Practical Professionalism in Medicine

A global case-based workbook

Edited by

ROGER WORTHINGTON

Independent Researcher, Policy Advisor and Medical Ethicist

and

RICHARD HAYS

Dean, Faculty of Health Sciences and Medicine
Bond University, Queensland, Australia

Illustrations by

DR ANDY WEARN

Associate Professor/Director
Clinical Skills Centre
The University of Auckland, New Zealand

Foreword by

PROFESSOR JIM McKILLOP

Emeritus Muirhead Professor of Medicine
University of Glasgow

Radcliffe Publishing
London • New York

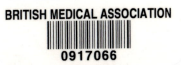

Radcliffe Publishing Ltd
33–41 Dallington Street
London
EC1V 0BB
United Kingdom

www.radcliffehealth.com

British Library Cataloguing in Publication Data

A catalogue record for this book is available from the British Library.

ISBN-13: 978 184619 584 6

The paper used for the text pages of this book is FSC® certified. FSC (The Forest Stewardship Council®) is an international network to promote responsible management of the world's forests.

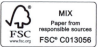

Typeset by Darkriver Design, Auckland, New Zealand
Printed and bound by TJI Digital, Padstow, Cornwall, UK

Contents

8 Postscript   171
   Roger Worthington and Richard Hays

Foreword

Professionalism is at the centre of the compact between the medical profession and the public and it underpins the trust that the public has in doctors.[1] It is of considerable topical interest and the subject of no little debate. Professional values have always influenced clinical practice, but the last 20 years or so have seen an increasing analysis of what constitutes medical professionalism, a feeling that it is under 'broad attack'[1] and calls for a change in the nature of professionalism.[2] Statements on the role of the doctor often emphasise the importance of professionalism,[3] and all too often medical disasters have lack of medical professionalism as at least a contributory factor.[4]

So why, then, is there so much debate about medical professionalism? A significant reason is the continuing disagreement about what exactly it covers and thus the lack of a widely agreed and precise definition. Professionalism clearly overlaps with fitness to practise (or 'fitness to serve' in the United States) but it is broader and more positive than that. Fitness to practise is concerned with assessing whether a particular doctor meets a minimum standard such that there can be reasonable assurance about the safety of patients in his or her care. Professionalism, by contrast, is about high standards and doing all that one can to constantly improve one's own performance. Professionalism also overlaps with ethics but, again, it is much broader. Matters involving professionalism can have ethical elements but may also be about other concerns, such as dealing with uncertainty or team-working.

Another area of debate is whether professionalism can be taught and assessed and what role it should have in medical curricula. In some countries (e.g. the four countries – Australia, New Zealand, the United States and the United Kingdom – from which the case studies in this book are drawn) it is firmly embedded in the curriculum for basic medical education.[5,6] There is legitimate debate about the best ways of teaching and assessing professionalism and there is recognition that a variety of approaches may be needed. However, in my view there is no excuse for not doing the best we can now in this area using the techniques we have available, while continually trying to improve on them. In other countries professionalism is largely absent from the medical curriculum. This matters because of the increasing internationalisation of medical education and the mobility of significant numbers of doctors. While there may be cultural reasons for professional values to vary from one country to another, a patient consulting a doctor has a right to expect that the doctor will be aware of and will abide by nationally agreed professional values wherever he or she has been educated.

Against this background, this book by Roger Worthington and Richard Hays is timely. They draw on a wealth of experience garnered in Australasia, the United Kingdom and North America. In the first part of the book they explore topics such as what constitutes professionalism; how it might best be taught and assessed; the interactions between professionalism, ethics and legal frameworks; international trends in medical education in relation to professionalism; and implications for public policy. These issues are explored in an open and very readable way. There is clear acknowledgement of areas of debate or lack of evidence. In their discussions, they provide a distillation of knowledge and information that anyone with an interest in the topic will find valuable. The second part of the book comprises around 30 case studies raising issues of professionalism involving medical students or doctors in training. These case studies are based on real cases and were compiled with the assistance of colleagues in the four countries concerned. Set out in a common format, these cases identify key discussion points for each scenario. They will be an invaluable resource for students and teachers alike.

I welcome this book unreservedly and I am sure it will play an important role in furthering the teaching of medical professionalism.

Professor Jim McKillop
Emeritus Muirhead Professor of Medicine
University of Glasgow
July 2013

REFERENCES

1. Working Party of the Royal College of Physicians. Doctors in society: medical professionalism in a changing world. *Clin Med.* 2005; 5(Suppl. 1): S5–40.
2. Smith R. Medical professionalism: out with the old and in with the new. *J R Soc Med.* 2006; 99(2): 48–50. Available at: www.ncbi.nlm.nih.gov/pmc/articles/PMC1360477 (accessed 4 April 2013).
3. Academy of Medical Royal Colleges, *et al. The Consensus Statement on the Role of the Doctor.* 2009. Available at: www.medschools.ac.uk/AboutUs/Projects/Documents/Role%20of%20Doctor%20Consensus%20Statement.pdf (accessed 4 April 2013).
4. *Report of the Mid Staffordshire NHS Foundation Trust Public Inquiry: executive summary.*

London: The Stationery Office; 2013. Available at: www.midstaffspublicinquiry. com/sites/default/files/report/Executive%20summary.pdf (accessed 4 April 2013).

5. General Medical Council. *Tomorrow's Doctors*. London: GMC; 2009. Available at: www.gmc-uk.org/education/undergraduate/tomorrows_doctors_2009.asp (accessed 4 April 2013).

6. General Medical Council; Medical Schools Council. *Medical Students: professional values and fitness to practise*. London: GMC; 2009. Available at: www.medschools. ac.uk/Publications/Documents/GMC_MedicalStudents.pdf (accessed 4 April 2013).

Preface

Professionalism is everyone's business in the world of twenty-first-century healthcare. It is no longer the case that professionalism is something that only scholars think about as a subject of theoretical inquiry. This is a workbook, and as authors we had two aims when we started writing, the first of which was to take the subject 'out of its box' and examine it in the cold light of day, stripped of any pretensions or exclusivity. While it is a privilege for someone to be able to claim the status of being a practising health professional, 'membership' is not an automatic right and members of any profession have to earn status through skill, hard work and acting responsibly.

It is fair to say that not all doctors behave professionally, or not all of the time, and when considering appropriate responses to *unprofessional* conduct one has to remember that doctors are human beings and so have their failings, and that sometimes these failings get in the way and prevent a doctor from doing his or her job safely and effectively. The public needs to know about this and to be aware that consequences follow when someone behaves unprofessionally, and responses to such behaviours should as far as possible be intelligent, fair and proportionate. Patients and the public deserve nothing less, and a doctor can similarly feel protected from knowing that the profession sets high standards and that when those standards are *not* met, some form of penalty is likely to follow.

On rare occasions this can suffice to cause someone to have to give up on long-held plans of becoming a doctor, or to give up on being allowed to remain in a responsible position that affects the lives of patients. At other times, the response is more nuanced and less final, depending on the particular circumstances of each case. By reading the cases, readers should be able to gain a sense of how things work in different settings and the range of issues that can arise – for example, when a doctor in training is found to be misusing drugs, is being dishonest or unreliable, or is entering into an inappropriate relationship.

The second reason for writing this book was to provide practical help to learners, teachers, programme leaders and healthcare institutions, and especially to help those in positions of responsibility to deal fairly and effectively with problems as and when they arise. Medical educators and regulatory bodies sometimes struggle when they are devising responses to complex and challenging situations. For this reason, two-thirds of this book comprises case studies taken from around the world and based on real life. We protect the identity of the individuals concerned and for this reason we fictionalise slightly, but nothing has been drawn from 'thin air'. Every case has elements of truth, and in each instance the subject is a trainee – either a doctor who is practising while still being trained or a medical student who is starting out on a journey that will eventually lead to him or her becoming a fully qualified medical professional. We recognise that some of the issues we discuss could apply equally to members of the other health professions; however, the object of our investigation is medicine and the difficulties that trainees can encounter on the journey towards becoming a fully qualified doctor.

The situations that we discuss in the narratives could similarly apply to more experienced members of the profession. However, in that instance the way in which a case might be handled could be different, so we restrict ourselves to doctors in training and draw on help that we received from senior, experienced medical educators around the world. This is a team effort, and while as authors we wrote the original material for the chapters, as well as some of the cases, as editors we are grateful to our contributing authors; however, we take ultimate responsibility for the full content, so any errors or omissions are ours and ours alone.

We hope that readers will find this book interesting, informative, useful and thought-provoking. The introductory chapters set the scene and discuss current issues, including matters of public policy, and we close by offering practical tips for educators and policymakers, together with analysis of some of the underlying trends that we identify through having worked on these issues for a number of years. The 'meat' in the middle of the sandwich is 29 in-depth case studies. While it will be for others to judge their merit, in our view the cases are never dull, and they can take the reader in some quite unexpected directions.

Roger Worthington
Richard Hays
July 2013

About the editors

Roger P Worthington MA, PhD, FAcadMed is an independent researcher, policy advisor and medical ethicist. Based in London, he holds honorary faculty positions at Yale University, Connecticut, and Bond University, Queensland, schools of medicine. He teaches ethics and professionalism to junior doctors in the NHS (UK) and is former subject lead on healthcare ethics and law at Keele University School of Medicine, England. He is a consultant advisor on workforce development at the Ministry of Health, New Zealand, and a former advisor on standards, ethics and education at the General Medical Council (UK).

Richard B Hays MBBS, PhD, MD, FRACGP is Dean of the Faculty of Health Sciences and Medicine at Bond University, Queensland, Australia. As a clinician, he works part-time as a general practitioner; his main academic interests are in curriculum and assessment design, programme evaluation and accreditation, and the measurement of professionalism. He lectures on these issues around the world and has ongoing quality assurance and advisory responsibilities with the medical regulator in the United Kingdom and in Australia. He has been instrumental in the establishment of new medical schools in Australia, Asia, Canada and Europe, including at Keele University in the United Kingdom.

List of contributors

Nancy Rockmore Angoff MD, MPH, MEd is Associate Dean for Student Affairs at Yale University School of Medicine and Associate Professor of Internal Medicine. As an attending physician at Yale-New Haven Hospital and the Nathan Smith Clinic at Yale, she specialises in the care of people with HIV/AIDS. Her interests include using literature to teach about medicine, teaching cultural awareness, medical ethics and the process of becoming a physician including development of a sense of professional identity. She has been a member of the Yale-New Haven Hospital Bioethics Committee since 1993.

Annette B Johnson BA, JD is Senior Vice President and General Counsel, New York University Hospitals Center, and Senior Counsel, NYU School of Medicine at NYU Langone Medical Center, where she has practised law as in-house counsel for 30 years. In these capacities, she provides legal advice and support to the governing board and executive leadership in all matters affecting academic medical centres, including academic advancement and processes for review of physicians and residents in regulatory matters.

Lynn Feldman Lowy BA, JD is Associate General Counsel at NYU Langone Medical Center. Prior to joining NYU Langone Medical Center she was an Assistant General Counsel in the legal department of Mount Sinai NYU Health. Previously, she was an associate in the healthcare department at the law firm Garfunkel, Wild & Travis, PC.

Jan McKenzie MBChB, FRCP (Can), FRANZCP is Associate Professor of Psychological Medicine and Associate Dean (Undergraduate Student Affairs) at the University of Otago, Christchurch. She is a member of the Fitness to Practise Committee of the Otago Medical School and a member of the New Zealand Health Practitioners' Disciplinary Tribunal.

Malcolm Parker MBBS, M Litt, M Hlth & Med Law, MD is Professor of Medical Ethics at the School of Medicine, University of Queensland. After being in general medical practice for over 30 years, he is now subject lead for ethics, law and professionalism on the Bachelor of Medicine/Bachelor of Surgery programme. He is a director of the Postgraduate Medical Council of Queensland, a member of the Health and Performance Committee of the Queensland Board of the Medical Board of Australia, and current president of the Australasian Association of Bioethics and Health Law.

Robert M Rohrbaugh MD is Professor of Psychiatry and Deputy Chair for Education and Career Development in the Department of Psychiatry at Yale University. His roles as Program Director in the Yale Psychiatry Residency Program, as a member of the Medical Student Progress Committee at Yale, and as a member of the Executive Committee of the American Association of Directors of Psychiatric Residency Training have provided him with substantial experience in the adjudication of professionalism issues in US medical trainees. Robert has experience with professionalism training in medical trainees in international settings through his roles as director of the Office of International Medical Student Education at Yale and as Visiting Professor at the Xiangya School of Medicine in Changsha, China.

Andy Wearn MBChB, MMedSc, MRCGP is Director of the Clinical Skills Centre at The University of Auckland. He moved to New Zealand in 2001, following an initial career in academic general practice in the United Kingdom. He is involved in undergraduate health professional programmes and postgraduate clinical education. In his spare time he channels his creativity through cooking and occasional artwork.

Daniel Weisberg BS is a medical student at Yale University School of Medicine, Connecticut. His first degree is from Brown University, Rhode Island, where he graduated Phi Beta Kappa, Magna Cum Laude, and with honours in biology. He plans to pursue a career in internal medicine with a focus on health policy. He has undertaken fellowships with the World Health Organization (Switzerland), Keele University (United Kingdom), and the Fellowship at Auschwitz for the Study of Professional Ethics programme (Poland).

Tim Wilkinson MBChB, M Clin Ed, MD, PhD, FRACP, FRCP is Professor in Medicine and Associate Dean (Medical Education) at the University of Otago, Christchurch. He chairs the Otago Faculty of Medicine Curriculum Committee and its assessment committee. His clinical work is in geriatric medicine, and his research interests are in assessment of clinical competence and performance, workplace learning, selection into medical school and professionalism.

Acknowledgements

We would like to express our thanks to each and every contributor. Without them there would be no book. The cases they provided were stimulating and exciting, and we say a big 'thank you' to Bob and Nancy; Annette and Lynn; Tim and Jan; Mal and Andy. We had three duos, where authorship of the cases was a shared experience. This not only helped (in all probability) with the writing and the difficulty of full schedules and limited time but also it helped the book by having their shared wisdom. Collaborations can be extremely fruitful, and this has certainly been the case in writing this book. A special thank you goes to Andy for providing the illustrations and lifting the material off the page and bringing it to life; also, we would like to note our appreciation of Daniel's contribution. He took time out from his medical studies to help with Part Two, and having the insights of a current trainee on which to draw proved to be a real asset. Finally, we express our thanks to Jim McKillop for agreeing to write the Foreword. He writes in a private capacity, as an academic and medical educator, and we were thrilled to hear from him when he wrote to say that he would be happy to take on this task. We value his thoughts, not simply because he has been in positions of leadership but because of his depth of understanding about the complex worlds of medical education and training.

Part One

Background and analysis

CHAPTER 1

Introduction

In this chapter we set out the rationale for this book, explaining why it was written, how the material is organised and how readers may want to use it.

PB, a 23-year-old final-year medical student, submits just before the deadline a clinical rotation/clerkship ITA (in-training assessment) form, signed by the clinical preceptor, stating that his performance has been satisfactory. However, the rotation/clerkship coordinator notices that while the signature has the same name as the preceptor's, a well-known senior clinician, the signature looks different. Aware of the possibility that it is a forgery, the rotation/clerkship coordinator refers the matter to the rotation/clerkship director, who calls PB in for an interview. When confronted with the different signatures PB admits to signing the form. He states that he had left the signing of the form until the last day and then could not find the preceptor; however, as he had been told that his performance was satisfactory, he had thought it acceptable to sign the form on behalf of the preceptor. The rotation/clerkship coordinator then contacts the preceptor, who confirms that PB's performance was indeed satisfactory but also states that he was not pleased PB had left the signing of the form to the last minute; the preceptor notes that 'PB had not tried very hard to find me, as I was in the hospital all day'.

Discussions about professionalism run the risk of raising more questions than they answer, because episodes of possible poor professionalism, such as in the case scenario given here, are often complex, raising issues that are open to interpretation more than providing clear-cut answers. In considering the cases that we provide in Part Two of this book it could be tempting to try to limit complexity by identifying single issues for discussion within each case. However, this would not make for interesting reading, and more than that, it would not reflect life. Cases involving unprofessional conduct often have several strands to them, and just as people have different facets to their character, so too do our subjects. At first glance the case at the opening of this chapter appears to concern a simple act of dishonesty, but after considering other issues something altogether more complex begins to emerge, and one's initial response may not be either 'right' or appropriate.

While it is comforting to find simple answers to simple questions, in our experience cases almost always have different layers, and one type of behaviour, for instance, could be masking another seemingly unrelated problem, or it could be involving a third party. Complexity adds interest but it also adds reality, and truth can indeed be stranger than fiction.

The question that must be asked before going any further in a discussion about professionalism is 'what *is* professionalism?' We recognise that medical professionalism is not a stable, easily defined construct, and while we address this issue more fully in Chapter 2, our aim is to provide an overview more than a comprehensive review of the subject as a whole. We offer this definition as a starting point:

> A profession may be described as a group that self-regulates, adopting processes and procedures that acknowledge members' training and individual responsibilities, recognising that their actions and behaviours could pose risks to the public that they seek to serve. Medical professionalism, therefore, is concerned with the standards of conduct that members of the profession (including those in training) should demonstrate in their day-to-day work.

Some people argue that professionalism in medicine has not changed since the days of Hippocrates, since from that era came the concepts of doing no harm to patients; applying scientific knowledge diligently and honestly; treating patients holistically, not as a collection of organs and symptoms; viewing other members of the profession as collaborative colleagues; and having regard for teaching as an essential or 'sacred' role. However, that is only part of the story, and while patients may still tend to regard doctors highly in terms of trustworthiness and reliability, much has changed in terms of the way in which medicine is practised. Concepts of professionalism evolve over time, and periodically attempts are made to try to give it a more stable definition.[1,2]

While the last 200 years have seen the rise of science and a more evidence-based approach to medicine, members of the public sometimes seek other types of care, perhaps turning to complementary or alternative health practitioners when orthodox medicine does not come up with 'answers'. Key to both types of medicine is good, reliable judgement, and while medical practice is increasingly dominated by expensive equipment used to analyse and treat a variety of disorders, judgement remains a core skill. We have here a heady, fluid mixture with elements of philosophy, science, technology, power, money, ethics, safety, healing, trustworthiness, justice, access, rights, responsibilities, career opportunities and success, and life and death itself. In combination, this provides a powerful backdrop against which professional behaviours need to be assessed.

The perfect system for delivering healthcare has yet to be found (and probably never will be), and from a political perspective, the medical profession is seen as having a high degree of power and influence, which doctors sometimes wield in order to show leadership and to influence arrangements in terms of how healthcare systems operate. This situation has the potential to give rise to conflicts of interest, and while the profession needs good leaders, there needs to be integrity in the process of providing healthcare, including transparency about whose interests are seen as being more important – the clinician's or those of the patient and the community. Professionalism covers all these things; it provides some form of agreed standard for measuring individual behaviours, and it also forms part of a backdrop against which modern medicine can be seen to be practised.

WHY A NEW BOOK ON PROFESSIONALISM, AND HOW DID IT COME ABOUT?

Books on professionalism do not always help busy clinicians who have to manage cases of possible poor professionalism while working with constant pressures on time. Some discussions in the literature are lengthy and theoretical, using language that is unfamiliar to clinicians. While reading the literature will for some people be edifying, such approaches rarely provide methods that can be applied to specific cases, let alone answers or practical solutions. On the other hand, it might be possible to condense these principles down to manageable proportions and write using a vocabulary that is readily accessible. One model for this can be found in manuals on differential diagnoses and drug prescribing of the sort that used to weigh down the pockets of junior doctors. However, for our purposes this is not satisfactory, as it offers a reductionist approach that oversimplifies situations, ignoring uncertainties and limiting the scope for the exercise of individual or collective judgement.

Medical professionalism has elements in common with other types of professionalism, and much of what we write could apply to other groups of professionals. Nonetheless, some topics concern doctors more than nurses and allied health professionals, for instance, and they may not be relevant to lawyers, accountants or other professionals at all. While some issues within medical professionalism may be considered universal, context and setting can make a difference. This could be on account of issues pertaining to one country or social setting as opposed to another, or having to do with one form of practical jurisprudence being adopted as opposed to another; however, the clinical element of care varies too, and it makes a difference what type of care is being provided by whom, when and where.

The examples we use in the cases that compose Part Two concern the *practice* of medicine, and we are not aware of other publications covering this ground in quite the same way; we aim to fill a gap in the literature with this case-based approach to medical professionalism. If this book helps one medical school create a more viable policy framework than might otherwise have been the case as regards fitness to practise (or progress), if one clinical teacher gains a better understanding of the issues, or if one doctor in training finds this practical approach helps him or her wrestle with challenges to *his or her* professional practice, then these efforts will have proved worthwhile. Anything beyond that will simply be a bonus. Medical practice changes one episode of care at a time, and while we are clearly interested in professional standards, we are not trying to *set* global standards or, for that matter, to revolutionise the practice of medicine (or anything else).

The editors have collaborated over a period of time, running workshops in different countries on responses to unprofessional conduct that is sometimes displayed by doctors in training. It can be challenging for committees and regulators to know how best to respond, in terms of either looking for remediation or the necessary imposition of sanctions. We think these topics are interesting, and delegates attending these workshops seemed to think so too. We have written about this subject elsewhere but have not previously produced anything as organised and systematic – hence this book.[3,4]

WHAT DOES THIS BOOK AIM TO ACHIEVE?

This book hopes to identify core elements of professionalism that apply in a range of settings involving medical professionals across the range in terms of professional experience, from early undergraduate through to postgraduate and continuing medical education. The authors want to see how common problems are addressed in different ways according to where problems arise. While there may be good reason for apparent inconsistencies, such as differences in legal systems or agreed ethical codes, differences can also serve to highlight weaknesses in local or national systems for addressing unprofessional conduct. This highlights the need to ensure equity and fairness in relation to disciplinary procedures for doctors in training, which is the group on which we focus in this book.

Questions of justice should not be avoided, and it is reasonable to ask why doctors are not treated fairly if the same 'offence' attracts a greater or lesser penalty in one school or one jurisdiction than another. Questions of fairness also arise in relation to protecting public interest; in other words, we ask if patients are being treated fairly, and if systems are fit for purpose, promoting a culture of safety and protecting the public from unprofessional and/or unsafe doctors. We do not wish to pretend that all unprofessional doctors are by definition unsafe; while there is a connection, saying there is a connection is different to saying there is an equivalence. What we do say is that unsafe doctors can pose a risk to patients by reason of their behaviour, which is a claim that we think *can* be upheld.

The future career of doctors is something that matters and is worth trying to save where possible (and appropriate), but it is not the only consideration, and public interest plays an important part in this debate. Through central taxation the public often makes a considerable investment in the training of doctors; in addition, and perhaps more important, if public interest is overlooked the result can spell disaster for future patients. Throughout this book we analyse professional problems from both of these perspectives. Poor governance can lead to poor clinical care, meaning that patients are harmed, occasionally even paying for it with their lives.[5] Professionalism is therefore something that governments and regulators need to take seriously; this is not a subject of 'mere' academic interest – it has a sharp edge, which we think ought perhaps to be better acknowledged.

HOW IS THIS BOOK ORGANISED (AND WHY)?

While there is little agreement about methodology when it comes to doing comparative analysis, we try to avoid some of the worst pitfalls, and when crossing continents various difficulties arise even where the language appears the same. While all cases originate from English-speaking countries, 'English' English and American English are not the same thing, and Australian English and New Zealand English have their own variants. Even if terminology can be agreed upon, frameworks and terms of reference change from one place to another.

You can substitute 'attending' for 'consultant' when referring to a senior, experienced clinician, but when the *way* doctors are trained varies so much in terms of structures and organisations (e.g. between the United States and the United Kingdom, or between states and territories), it becomes evident that differences are not just about language. Cultural and structural differences also play a part, and when planning this book we came to the pragmatic view that it made better sense to bracket cases into two main groups: (1) the United States and the United Kingdom and (2) Australia and New Zealand. We do not wish to ignore our colleagues in Canada, or in any other country where English is the dominant language; we simply take a practical view that limits have to be set, and that on account of personal connections and direct experience, these countries will be the focus of our attention. Spreading the net further would make the project too unwieldy and would risk causing confusion.

Chapter 2 is where we share our thoughts on relevant theories underpinning the practical decisions that have to be made when looking at individual cases; this is where we address terminology, discuss definitions and review the literature. This also includes educational issues around learning and teaching and different methods of assessment. We make no attempt to say *how* the subject should be taught or to provide model exam questions, since the *cases* are what make up the practical component of this book. The setting of exam questions is a topic for another day (or another team of authors).

Chapter 3 is where ethical considerations take centre stage, and where more philosophical elements arising from the case are discussed in greater detail than would be appropriate within the context of the cases studies. We do not favour the traditional 'four principles' approach to medical ethics; in our view that approach is too narrow and lacks practical value. This does not stop us from talking about justice and autonomy, for instance, but we tend to favour the language of rights as having greater applicability to the type of situations we encounter.

Chapter 4 is about medical education and international trends. We address issues such as the globalisation of medicine, multiculturalism and societal change, and the aging of society. We also tackle some jurisdictional and cultural differences affecting medical education and practice in the countries covered by the cases in Part Two. We go on to consider the practical matter of how students are selected for entry into medical school, because without that, the whole conversation about medical professionalism could be wrong-footed. If selection processes are inadequate, one could end up with a workforce that is different from the one that was first envisaged – for instance, when setting up a new school of medicine.*

Chapter 5 is where we focus on public policy implications of medical professionalism, and what it means when things go wrong. Major scandals occasionally hit the headlines when doctors behave in such a shocking way as to cause questions to be asked in parliament. We discuss ethical and policy issues around medical regulation and workforce planning, including the revalidation of doctors, which after 20 years of planning became a practical reality

---

* This is something that RH has done more than once; he speaks from direct experience but without claiming to be an authority on this complex and multifaceted task.

in the United Kingdom during the period of time when this book was being written.

Fitness to practise, or fitness to progress, is a matter of considerable relevance to trainee doctors, and medical students or junior doctors whose behaviour is deemed unprofessional should expect to be sanctioned in some way. The range of sanctions starts with somebody having additional supervision or having to retake a year at medical school and moves all the way up to career-breaking episodes where somebody will be prevented from graduating or working in clinical practice. In between these two ends of the spectrum are various gradations, and medical educators will be aware that a small number of students and trainees will have to face disciplinary hearings of some kind. The nuances of these issues are discussed in the cases, where local context helps to provide meaning and relevance.

Part Two makes up the bulk of this book, and we present a range of cases taken from real life, although modified in order to protect the identity of the individuals and institutions concerned. We value the cases we received from our team of experienced and distinguished contributing authors and are grateful for their efforts. *Chapter 6* covers cases from the United Kingdom and the United States, while *Chapter 7* covers cases from Australia and New Zealand. The format of each case is consistent, starting with an outline, followed by a short list of questions arising from the case; next comes the discussion section, and the presented case ends with a summary of key points in the form of answers to standardised questions (as listed at the beginning of *Chapter 6*).

For readers wanting to read the cases straight through, the step-by-step sequence should be easy to follow, and in determining the order of cases we have loosely bracketed them together. For instance, in *Chapter 6* we start with all the cases relating to drug misuse, and in *Chapter 7* we begin with cases that have a mental health component, followed in both instances by cases involving other types of behavioural problems, including poor clinical performance. In *Chapter 8* we draw things together and consider findings that can be extrapolated from the cases as a whole, such as how and why some topics occur more frequently than others. We close by offering a 10-point plan as a guide to teachers and learners and hope that in sharing some difficulties that arise when doctors have problems with professionalism this will help to promote best practice in medical education and training. This is one way of helping to protect patients from unsafe doctors.

RESPONDING TO UNPROFESSIONAL BEHAVIOURS IS OFTEN DIFFICULT: WHY?

While the answer to the question 'why is responding to unprofessional behaviours often difficult' will be made clearer later on, it is worth identifying here some potential difficulties than can arise.

1. *Weaknesses in systems and procedures*: if policies and procedures are unclear or inconsistent, they will be difficult to follow and may not stand up under the pressure of scrutiny (e.g. when lawyers become involved).
2. *Regulatory frameworks might be weak, unclear or even non-existent*: educators may be perfectly willing to follow guidance but there needs to be consistency, which is difficult to achieve if frameworks are inadequate or missing.
3. *Few cases are open and shut*: judgement has to be exercised in making decisions, based on the merits of each case. Acknowledging grey areas is one thing, but being able to form judgements when the facts are uncertain and/ or where there is an element of moral ambiguity is something else.
4. *It is often assumed that there is an association between academic ability and professionalism, such that superior academic ability can 'compensate' for poor professionalism*. However, there is little evidence for this assertion, and judgement about the behaviour of individuals should be made independently of academic performance.
5. *Mitigating circumstances*: sometimes cases present with plausible explanations that could count as mitigation; doctors in training may try to explain their actions, but they may not have insight into why their behaviours were considered inappropriate.
6. *Deciding penalties*: having reached a decision about wrongdoing, deciding on appropriate sanctions or penalties can be as difficult as reaching the decision in the first place. Details depend on context and jurisdiction, but the parameters for determining fair and proportionate responses need to be clearly defined and properly addressed.
7. *Predicting future patterns based on past behaviour*: this is speculative and not an exact science; those charged with making decisions about others need to bear this in mind. Being too lenient may harm future patients but being too harsh may be unjust to trainees, neither course of action being desirable.[6]

TEACHING AND ASSESSING PROFESSIONALISM: A USEFUL EXERCISE OR A WASTE OF TIME?

While we will talk about teaching and assessment in *Chapter 2*, we do not ask the rather basic question of 'why bother?' Perhaps it is because we have an interest in these issues and therefore assume it is pointless to ask this question; or perhaps it is because we figure that you are already reading this book and have shown an interest, hence the question is already redundant. However, there is a point that needs making, which is not made elsewhere; namely, that *not* all countries and systems of medical education and training hold the subject of medical professionalism in equal esteem (i.e. affording it equal priority with other topics as regards space and time in the curriculum). In some countries the model for practising medicine is still paternalistic, and the idea that patients have rights may be considered novel or just irrelevant (which plainly is not a view that we hold); this may well be the case in developing countries, especially in public hospitals.[7] Furthermore, some people could argue that 'it's pointless to try to teach professionalism, because it comes about simply through example, and through students and trainees being immersed in the culture of medicine'. We agree that role modelling matters and that it influences students and trainees, but we do not believe these influences are always good, or that they mean professionalism should *not* be given time and space in the curriculum.

Doctors often move from one country to another, and there are plenty of doctors in training whose primary education occurred in a different country to the one in which they currently work and train. For these people the model of professionalism with which they grew up may be different from the one that is now expected. Cultural conditioning is a fact of life, and we cannot ignore the fact that some people's ideals reflect a form of cultural conditioning that may not mesh with the cultural norms that apply to the host country. Nonetheless, ethical and legal requirements come into play, and doctors have to adhere to local guidelines, which can sometimes lead to tension between local expectations (i.e. in terms of professional behaviours that would be seen as normal in other settings).

With this workbook we adopt an approach that does not seek to limit complexity or uncertainty. While we try to avoid leaving loose ends hanging in the air, this does not imply that straightforward answers to complex questions are just there waiting to be found. In the context of medical education, issues arising are sometimes *more* complicated than in ordinary clinical practice, because learners are on a path falling somewhere between 'novice' or 'proto-professional' and 'experienced professional'.[8] This could be seen to justify a claim such that trainees are somehow less responsible by reason of their lack of experience, but this reasoning does not follow and may not count as a mitigating factor.

In addressing these matters we aim to make the subject accessible, leaning towards the practical side of the theory-versus-practice equation. While this book should be useful to educators with roles in teaching professionalism and/or managing possible poor professionalism in learners and trainees, our intention is for this book to have a wider appeal, and certainly to include health professionals in training. Furthermore, the public has a right to know the type of issues that arise and how such matters are addressed.

In short, this book is about medical professionalism in workplace and educational settings, and it is about considering appropriate responses to unprofessional behaviours, taking account of public interest, patient safety and the need to promote equity and justice. Readers can decide whether or not we have succeeded in this endeavour.

REFERENCES

1. Levenson R, Dewar S, Shepherd S; Royal College of Physicians. *Understanding Doctors: harnessing professionalism*. London: King's Fund; 2008. Available at: www.kingsfund. org.uk/publications/understanding-doctors (accessed 2 May 2013).
2. Royal College of Physicians. *Future Physician: changing doctors in changing times; report of a working party*. London: RCP; 2010. Available at: http://bookshop.rcplondon. ac.uk/details.aspx?e=314 (accessed 8 February 2013).
3. Worthington R, Hays R. Responding to unprofessional behaviours. *Clin Teach*. 2011; 9(2): 71–4.
4. Hays R, Hamlin G, Worthington R. Developing professionalism in health professional learners. *Clin Teach*. 2013; 10(1): 64–6.
5. Van Der Weyden MB. The Bundaberg Hospital scandal: the need for reform in Queensland and beyond. *Med J Aust*. 2005; 183(6): 284–5.
6. Papadakis MA, Teherani A, Banach MA, *et al*. Disciplinary action by medical boards and prior behavior in medical school. *New Engl J Med*. 2005; 353(25): 2673–82.
7. Worthington RP. Medicine, ethics and professionalism in modern India. In: Worthington RP, Rohrbaugh RM. *Health Policy and Ethics: a critical examination of values from a global perspective*. London: Radcliffe Publishing; 2011. pp. 72–5.
8. Hilton SR, Slotnick HB. Proto-professionalism: how professionalisation occurs across the continuum of medical education. *Med Educ*. 2005; 39(1): 58–65.

CHAPTER 2

Professionalism

While this chapter talks about definitions and concepts, we try here to dispel some of the myths surrounding professionalism, we consider the subject from different angles and we conclude with a section on the education and assessment of future doctors.

Now is the time to consider what we mean by the term 'professionalism'. We are not concerned so much with finding the best definition as we are with discussing relevant concepts and considering their application, which is a slightly different task. People may profess to know what is meant by professionalism; however, ask health professionals to describe professionalism and they might not find it so easy. Using negative descriptions would be one way to respond, by saying what professionalism is *not*, but this approach has its limitations, since if professionalism is only recognisable by its absence, the implication is that nobody knows what it is. Furthermore, simply describing behaviour as being either 'professional' or 'unprofessional' is circular, unless there is a degree of clarity about what these terms mean. Without examining the concept and its application it is difficult to get beyond the actual words, leaving one without a response to the assertion sometimes made that *'you know professionalism when you see it'*. By this analysis unprofessionalism would have to be behaviour that does not conform to agreed norms, and this line of reasoning has more promise than the purely negative definition.

If professionalism is about 'what *not* to do' or, worse still, if it is simply code for 'do as *I* do', then the expression has little value. Lying and cheating, for example, would not be listed as types of behaviours that would be expected from a practising health professional, but, as doctors are human beings, occasionally these behaviours will occur; when they do, one needs an appropriate response.

To adopt a positive stance, suitable keywords for professionalism could include *understanding, insight, honesty, patience, empathy*, and so forth. In addition, phrases such as *being accountable, being disciplined, showing good judgement, acting responsibly, having regard to the needs of others, showing respect for patients, demonstrating competence and skill, having integrity, inspiring trust*, and so forth, have their uses. However, even this does not take us very far, since most of these words or phrases could be applied to someone who does *not* work as a medical or other professional (or, for that matter, someone who does not work at all). Therefore, one can select and combine words and phrases that have relevance to a clinician going about his or her daily work, but what about when they're off duty? The clinician is still a professional and to some extent has to conform to certain standards; therefore, phrases and expressions only applicable in the workplace have limited practical value.

THE CONCEPT

In terms of concepts and applications of the term 'professionalism', we argue that it applies to *persons* rather than the behaviours they exhibit. This avoids the pitfalls of circularity and subjectivity from being limited by descriptive words and phrases. It is *people* who behave or misbehave, and it is *persons* (people) who display attributes such as those required to ensure that a patient is able to trust his or her physician. Attributes influence behaviours, so if we choose to examine models of professional behaviour, it is important to consider the sum of the parts, asking 'who is the *person* inside the white coat?' (That is, if anyone still wears one.)

By this reasoning, if a person has sound judgement, he or she is less likely to behave unprofessionally than someone who externally appears to be thoroughly professional but whose behaviour is unpredictable or unreliable. However, arguing that personal attributes are important gives rise to the question of 'if and how they should be acquired, learned or taught', to which we will return later. To summarise, so far we have established that primarily the concept of professionalism is one that concerns *persons, attributes* and *behaviours* – in that order.

Next we come to the question of application, which has considerable relevance, since people often define themselves by making reference to what they do and where. By focusing on application we draw attention to what doctors *do* as opposed to what they are *supposed* to do; that is, provide an appropriate standard of clinical care in a way that poses minimal risk to the public, while earning respect and trust from patients as well as colleagues. This way one can come a little closer to identifying values and attributes that might be expected from a practising professional. We consistently argue that professional behaviours acquire meaning by virtue of their application. One does not have to be a practising professional to work hard, keep high standards and work well with colleagues, but attributes such as these take on added meaning when considered in relation to the context or setting in which they apply. It matters greatly what you do, where you do it and how, and a person with the right attributes should be able to demonstrate that they are meeting the standards expected of them both in and out of the workplace. We do not believe that professionalism is something you can just turn on and off.

In short, professionalism concerns the person, and one does not cease to be that person the moment one leaves the workplace. If 'following protocol' is all there is to being a doctor then it would not require 10 years of training in order to be properly qualified.

There is a substantial body of literature on professionalism, which we encourage readers to explore.[1-4] While we could easily spend 100 pages working through this literature and adding our own judgements and observations, we refer to (rather than review) works in the literature in preference to trying to provide a comprehensive overview. For example, we draw the reader's attention to a much-cited literature review (1982–2002) on assessing professionalism,[5] a paper summarising results from a systematic review matching assessment tools to definable elements in professionalism[6] and a paper challenging monocultural Western models of professionalism.[7]

PROFESSIONALISM AND PUBLIC POLICY

Periodically, the medical profession comes under especially close scrutiny, usually following a scandal or a high-profile case that was brought to public attention via the media. Governments and public bodies have to be *seen* to be responding, and there is a political side to professionalism that should not be overlooked. Putting aside questions relating to healthcare delivery and reform that fall outside the scope of this book, it is not difficult to see why medical professionalism sometimes becomes a matter of public policy. For this reason, we afford it a special chapter and refer readers to Chapter 5 for a fuller discussion about this side of professionalism.

In the context of this chapter, we provide an example of a public scandal arising out of a case of professionalism that was of such a low standard as to lead to a public investigation and to the doctor in question being sent to jail. We refer to the Australian case of a surgeon, Dr Jayant Patel, who worked for Queensland Health. Here, an issue that became a matter of public confidence arose when a surgeon with a long history of poor clinical outcomes came to be appointed director of surgery at a public hospital north of Brisbane.[8] Dr Patel, prior to being offered an appointment, failed to disclose material facts relating to him having being prevented from performing surgical procedures when practising in the United States. What made matters worse was that his employer (Queensland Health) and the regulator (The Medical Board of Queensland), appear not to have performed adequate background checks before confirming his appointment, simply taking his word at face value. His lack of competence and lack of probity became highly corrosive when coupled with inefficiencies in local administration and reluctance on the part of senior managers to face up to what was going on. This state of affairs seriously undermined the profession, and it echoed its way back to the Minister for Health; more significantly, it may have led to patients being maimed and to unnecessary, avoidable deaths, and so the consequences of this failure in professional standards could not have been more serious.[9]* As this book goes to press, the consequences of this case are still the subject of legal action.

In Chapter 5, in the context of public policy and medical regulation, we refer to the case of Dr Harold Shipman in the United Kingdom and to the public inquiry into multiple killings carried out by this registered family physician over a 25-year period. The inquiry report ran to six volumes, the implications of which challenged the basic principle of medical self-regulation in the United Kingdom.[10] This scandal gave rise to a set of choices: (1) for government to step in and set up new regulatory frameworks and procedures or (2) for regulatory reforms to be undertaken, which is what did eventually happen, and the reforms are ongoing. Allowing the status quo to continue was never an option.

Dr Shipman's conduct was overtly criminal and profoundly unprofessional, yet reputedly he was much liked by his patients.† One of the main underlying problems seems to have been the repeated failure by Dr Shipman and others to recognise and address long-standing mental health problems. This situation was coupled with serious professional irregularities (e.g. in regard to arrangements for reporting deaths) that took place over a long period of time, resulting in Dr Shipman being allowed to carry on and cause hundreds of deaths. As can be seen in some of the cases in Part Two, health issues and professionalism issues are often linked, which is something that educators need to bear in mind. However, when a whole system fails, the social contract arrangement for medical regulation begins to fall apart.

Regulators set out the standards that are expected of a practising professional, either in a detailed, systematic way, as with the General Medical Council

---

* Sadly for the person who took great personal risk in exposing Dr Patel's incompetence, she had to wait 7 years before receiving financial compensation for the worry and stress that she had to go through after trying to 'blow the whistle'. Instead of being listened to she was threatened with losing her job, and it was not until a national paper took up the case that anyone began to pay attention to what she had been saying.

† RW has met former patients of Dr Shipman, and there are people living in Greater Manchester who miss having Dr Shipman as their general practitioner, even knowing what happened. For those unfamiliar with these events, Dr Shipman was tried and convicted for murder, and while in prison he took his own life.

in the United Kingdom,[11] or via other means. For instance, in Sweden, where medical regulation is a function of the state,[12] there are no such detailed guidelines other than those issued by the medical societies and colleges.[13] However professional guidelines are derived, practitioners need to know what the standards are and stick to them, and if there are no consequences for failing to meet those standards, then that could be considered a failure in public policy. It really is that simple, in principle, even if practical applications of ethical and professional standards are a little more complicated.

PROFESSIONALISM AND PATIENT CARE

The enterprise of upholding standards of professionalism is primarily for the purpose of promoting better standards of patient care. It may be difficult to *prove* the causal link between professionalism and quality patient care, but unless professionalism translates into better patient care it could be seen as just so much hot air, unless one takes the view that professionalism is an absolute value in and of itself. Given earlier comments that it is the *applications* of professionalism that really matter, we do not lend support to positions of absolutism. Rather, we argue that professionalism is about people – the type of person a medical practitioner is, and how he or she treats patients and has regard for '*the person in the patient*'.[14] While links between cause and effect in professional care and patient outcomes are sometimes notable by their absence, the quality of life that a patient leads after a medical intervention is important and deserves our attention. No form of treatment can ever guarantee quality of life, but quality of life should be considered when decisions are being made about the appropriateness of certain types of treatment; that is simply part of good professional practice. Quality of life also matters in routine situations, where a family physician, for instance, agrees a course of action that satisfies the needs and expectations of the patient.

To summarise, in order for a doctor to be professional, the doctor should be able to demonstrate (1) that he or she behaves appropriately, (2) that he or she knows what he or she is doing and keeps his or her knowledge and training up to date, (3) that he or she has listened to the patient and made an effort to understand the patient's needs and (4) that decisions not only involve the patient but also are made directly by the patient (if the patient has capacity). Physicians have to be able to communicate with their patients, have regard for patients' needs and wishes and, wherever possible, provide appropriate quality care. This is what is important about professionalism: *it makes a difference to patient care.*

ETHICS VERSUS PROFESSIONALISM

For the student or trainee, applied ethics is where professionalism in action starts to become a practical reality. However, first we need to consider an important distinction, determining when something is a matter of ethics and when it is primarily a matter of professionalism. The terms relate but they are not interchangeable, and we take the view that professionalism is the broader term and that ethics is the major subset. However, there may not be a consensus on this point, and in the United States, for instance, the term 'professionalism' is applied somewhat differently from the way it is used in a European context.*

To some, ethics is a philosophical discipline far more than it is a practical tool to be applied in a setting such as healthcare. To others, it can be argued (perhaps convincingly) that professionalism covers the whole way in which medicine is practised, and that ethics refers more to the moral dimensions of the enterprise. Not all aspects of clinical practice give rise to ethical problems or explicitly cause moral judgements to have to be made; however, in applied medical ethics, professionalism is a central tenet, and ethical considerations inform almost every aspect of how medicine is practised. Indeed, to consider the ethical dimensions of medicine without taking account of the professional context within which care is delivered would be an exercise with fairly limited value.

Clearly, ethical reasoning can be considered without any reference to a medical setting, and the history of philosophy has a long line of ethical writings, stretching from Aristotle to John Stuart Mill and others, none of whom address the practice of medicine. The converse is also true and self-evident – only some medical literature pertains to the subject ethics; therefore, the categories of ethics and professionalism interconnect at many different levels but they do not fall into the same intellectual space.

Imagine concentric circles: either ethics could be a circle within a circle, with professionalism on the outside, which we think is reasonable in an applied setting, or the two circles could overlap, which permits the possibility of intellectual inquiry into one domain without the other, and without one being subsumed into the other, which is probably more sustainable as a theoretical position. Because this book is about practice, not theory, we favour the first analogy over the second; we do not, however, argue that the alternative explanation is wrong – it just does not fit our present purpose.

To take a practical example, the General Medical Council in the United Kingdom publishes guidelines on standards and ethics: essentially, these guidelines are about professionalism and the way in which medicine is practised,

---

* For example, for many years Yale School of Medicine had a first-year course entitled 'Professional Responsibility'; however, topics covered by this course could be included in an introduction to medical ethics in different educational settings.

and only sometimes do they directly concern morals.* Guidelines on confidentiality, for instance, are about ethics, and yet respect for the principle of confidentiality is one of the oldest tenets of medical professionalism dating back to the time of Hippocrates; hence, in reality the matter is far from settled.[15]

Ethical values inform professional practice, and while that does not make it a truism that ethics and professionalism are inseparable, how a term is used over time influences that term's definition. While we define professionalism partly in relation to its ethical content, we make no claim to having the last word on this highly contentious issue; instead, we ask readers to keep an open mind on when and how to use the terms 'ethics' and 'professionalism', to be wary of false assumptions, and to try to avoid ambiguous use of terminology (which is not that easy).

PROGRESSION AND FITNESS TO PRACTISE

An expression that occurs repeatedly in the literature on professionalism (and used in some countries but not in others) is 'fitness to practise' (or 'practice', to give the verb its American English spelling). In other words, by using the expression, one is attempting to answer the question: 'Is a doctor a fit and proper person to be allowed to continue to practise medicine or to progress to the next level of training?' We return to this theme in Chapter 5, where there is an emphasis on public policy, but here the focus remains on professionalism and the consequences for individuals when things do not go as planned and someone steps out of line.

If a registered doctor or doctor in training behaves in a manner that is incompatible with being allowed to continue training or to practise medicine without restrictions, then it would be said that the doctor's fitness to practise has become *impaired*. However, in order to establish the nature and degree of impairment, judgement has to be formed first on whether or not the lapse in standards amounts to serious professional misconduct. In other words, when deciding serious professional misconduct a conclusion needs to be reached as to the extent of someone's impairment, which means reviewing the actions of the doctor or trainee. The outcome of that review could be the imposition of one of a number of different sanctions, including deregistration or being expelled from a programme, which could mark the end of someone's medical career, even before it has begun. Not all cases are so serious, and lesser sanctions can be put in place that are less far-reaching, but that depends on the issue in question, the nature of the individual case and where the case takes place.

---

* Ethics and morals are synonyms, although by application, ethics is the more widely used term in the context of medicine.

While similar issues arise with doctors and trainees in countries such as the United States, the process and the terminology are not the same. For example, in the United States, *progression* from one stage to the next is the expression normally used when considering whether or not someone's performance or professional standard has become impaired. Progression is indeed an important concept, especially in the educational setting, and in the event of a negative judgement being formed, for instance, that could mean a medical student or junior doctor having to resit an examination or undergo additional training.

There is another point to consider here, relating to the function and constitution of relevant committees. A progress committee in one institution, for instance, could be focusing on academic achievement whereas in another it could consider issues of probity and professionalism – that is, behaviours rather than intellectual ability or attainment – although in reality the two are often linked. Institutions will have to have suitable committees in place, staffed by suitably qualified members of the medical faculty, and in addition, there has to be a mechanism for appealing decisions made at school or programme level. However, there is no uniformity in terms of what these committees are called or how they relate to one another.*

This plurality of structures means there is lack of conformity between schools, states and medical systems, which can lead to inconsistent outcomes for otherwise similar lapses in professional conduct. While this situation is perhaps unavoidable, taking account of institutional autonomy, questions of legal jurisdiction and political independence, the range of behaviours exhibited by doctors will be similar around the world, and concepts of justice and ethical consistency need to be considered. Behaviours and academic achievement are both important in professional settings, and instances where trainees achieve good grades but give cause for concern on account of their attitudes, behaviours and/or perceived lack of insight can occur anywhere.[16] Adjudication in such cases is difficult, wherever it happens, and for this reason, we explore these issues more fully in Part Two.

TEACHING PROFESSIONALISM

Professionalism is now widely regarded as an essential and substantial component of medical curricula both at undergraduate and at postgraduate and specialty training levels. Gone are the days when medical curricula only covered the biomedical sciences, and clinical practice and 'clever' doctors were accepted even if they were not approachable or they did not have any understanding

---

* In the case studies presented in this book, we use local phraseology and respect local differences that relate to matters of jurisprudence; to do otherwise would probably be incoherent – terminology and process cannot be expected to conform across national or international borders.

about patient care. Doctors must now be not only scientists but also good communicators, with an understanding of the relevant healthcare system, thereby assisting patients to navigate a complex system and participate in their own care, whatever the setting or location in which the care is being provided. Furthermore, a substantial proportion of complaints against doctors relate to poor communication rather than poor knowledge or technical skill.[17] Doctors facing disciplinary charges mid-career sometimes have a record of unprofessional behaviours stemming from their student days,[18] strengthening the current view that professionalism should and probably can be taught.

Contemporary approaches to medical education still have a major focus on the scientific basis of medical practice, but this has been extended to include behavioural and social sciences – particularly, interpersonal communication and how healthcare systems function. Issues such as leadership; legal and ethical frameworks; accountability; respect for patients, peers and self; and understanding one's limits are (or ought to be) addressed early, regularly and throughout medical curricula. Furthermore, admissions processes often include consideration of professionalism issues during the selection process, ensuring that learners are aware they are joining a profession that comes with special responsibilities *prior* to enrolment on the course.

Curricula are typically organised *horizontally* into subjects or phases and *vertically* into domains or themes. Both organisational structures can facilitate integration of content within and across academic years towards achievement of the knowledge, skills and attitudes required by the completion of the programme. This results in improved contextualisation of learning (horizontal integration) and development, building on content that was provided during each academic year. One common approach is to regard the roles of doctors as one of the curriculum themes, an example of which can be found in the UK General Medical Council's three-theme model of the doctor as *scholar* and *scientist*, *practitioner* and *professional*, as established in *Tomorrow's Doctors*.[19]

There may be no single best way of teaching professionalism to health professionals. While it is true that professionalism topics can, and probably should, be covered in a variety of teaching and learning methods – lectures, tutorials, seminars, problem-based learning case discussions, and debates within clinical placements and clinical case presentations – these methods form the *planned* curriculum rather than the *delivered* curriculum. That is, learners often have learning experiences that are not necessarily intended or even recognised. The gap between the planned and the delivered curriculum is the *hidden* curriculum: the most powerful components here are observation of poor professionalism by individual clinicians and poor patient experiences when patients are 'caught' in the healthcare system and do not receive the idealised model of care that is espoused in the medical curriculum.

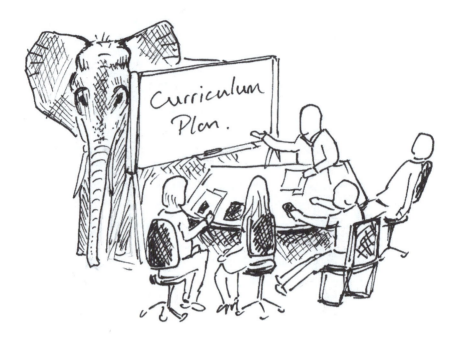

Role modelling can be an extremely powerful influence, but clinical teachers have been known to display similar poor behaviours to the learners who are attached to them.[20] Medical students all too easily model poor behaviours, thereby replicating standards of professional conduct that one would not want them to emulate.

Replicating poor professional practice will never be good for patients and the public; but more than that, it is bad for medical student and junior doctor morale. If a young doctor aspires to 'do things better', it is highly demoralising to find that 'nothing changes' in terms of behaviours that are observed and tolerated, including from one's peers. The line of least resistance can be simply to follow suit because 'it's too difficult trying to bring about change'. Not only does it take energy, commitment and a willingness to follow through to bring about a change in the professional culture but also it takes willingness on the part of those in senior positions to embrace and implement change. This rarely comes about quickly – it could even take a generation.

ASSESSING PROFESSIONALISM

We have noted that there is potentially a gap between the planned and the delivered curriculum, and if the assessment of learners is not carefully aligned with learning outcomes then learners may be assessed on material that is either not planned or not delivered, but which nonetheless appears in examinations. Learners quickly hear about and share with one another what is in

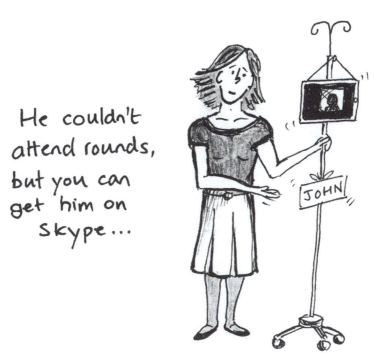

He couldn't attend rounds, but you can get him on Skype...

examinations, and so they naturally tend to study for the assessed curriculum focusing on past papers rather than having regard for the curriculum as a whole. It is essential, therefore, that the assessment of professionalism reflects what learners actually need to be learning.

Because professionalism is a broad topic that includes a range of quite different attributes, including attitudes and behaviours, it is important that assessment involves multiple methods, multiple judges and multiple occasions (early and often) over the duration of the training programme.[21] Multiple methods are required because the quite distinct attributes need to be assessed differently; for example, knowledge can be assessed in written tests; interpersonal communication can be observed in objective structured clinical examination stations; and teamwork, interprofessional collaboration and ethical conduct can be observed over time in the 'real' clinical environment. While many currently available methods can be used to assess professionalism,[5] others are being developed or adapted specifically to assess certain attributes, such as 360-degree evaluations, which are ideal for team-working and leadership attributes.[22]

The primary reason for assessing professionalism is to guide learning. Most educators would believe that learners have to develop knowledge of the cultures of healthcare and the health professions, and if errors are made, learners need to be able to learn from those errors. There is of course another potential purpose: if a learner is found to have persistent unprofessional behaviours, especially behaviours that do not respond to remediation, then the career of this learner is being put at risk. This more disciplinary component to assessing professionalism is a recurring theme, which we address in Part Two; the whole process requires careful documentation and for clear regulations to be in place (and followed) in order to try to ensure a smooth line of progression through medical education and training.

Summary

- It is *people* who behave (or misbehave); it is *people* who display attributes such as those required to ensure that patients feel able to trust their physician.
- *Professionalism* is not just an abstract concept; it affects patient care (as well as medical careers).
- Professionalism covers the whole way in which medicine is practised; *ethics*, however, refers to the moral dimensions of the enterprise.
- Not all aspects of clinical practice cause moral judgements to have to be made, but in *applied* medical ethics professionalism is a central tenet.
- Ethical considerations inform almost every aspect of *how* medicine is practised.
- Professionalism may seem impersonal and remote but it can't be ignored; some liken it to electricity – everybody needs it but you notice it most when it's *not* there.[23]
- Altruism versus self-interest – which prevails and when? This is a moral question with professional implications, and one that has to be considered every time a student or trainee faces a challenging situation in navigating a path between meeting clinical obligations, having a home life, and getting signed-off by a supervisor or appraiser and progressing to the next stage.
- Professionalism needs to be fully integrated into degree or training programmes; it should be assessed at different stages using various methods of assessment.

REFERENCES

1. Wear D, Aultman JM, editors. *Professionalism in Medicine: critical perspectives*. New York: Springer-Verlag; 2006.
2. Parsi K, Sheehan MN, editors. *A Medical Professionalism Primer*. Oxford: Rowman and Littlefield; 2006.

3. Thistlethwaite J, Spencer J. *Professionalism in Medicine.* Oxford: Radcliffe Publishing; 2008.

4. Kanes C, editor. *Elaborating Professionalism: innovation and change in professional education.* New York: Springer; 2010.

5. Lynch DC, Surdyk PM, Eiser AR. Assessing professionalism: a review of the literature. *Med Teach.* 2004; **26**(4): 366–73.

6. Wilkinson TJ, Wade WB, Knock LD. A blueprint to assess professionalism: results of a systematic review. *Acad Med.* 2009; **84**(5): 551–8.

7. Ho MJ, Yu KH, Hirsh D, *et al.* Does one size fit all? Building a framework for medical professionalism. *Acad Med.* 2011; **86**(11): 1407–14.

8. Van Der Weyden MB. The Bundaberg Hospital scandal: the need for reform in Queensland and beyond. *Med J Aust.* 2005; **183**(6): 284–5.

9. Thomas H. *Sick to Death: a manipulative surgeon and a health system in crisis; a disaster waiting to happen.* Sydney: Allen and Unwin; 2010.

10. Department of Health. *Shipman Inquiry Sixth Report.* London: Her Majesty's Stationery Office; 2005. Available at: http://webarchive.nationalarchives.gov.uk/20060715141954/http://the-shipman-inquiry.org.uk/home.asp (accessed 3 May 2013).

11. General Medical Council. *Duties of a Doctor.* London: GMC; 2013. Available at: www.gmc-uk.org/guidance/good_medical_practice/duties_of_a_doctor.asp (accessed 3 May 2013).

12. www.socialstyrelsen.se/english

13. www.sls.se/Om-SLS/In-English/

14. Goodrich J, Cornwell J. *Seeing the Person in the Patient.* London: King's Fund; 2009. Available at: www.kingsfund.org.uk/publications/the_point_of_care.html (accessed 30 January 2013).

15. General Medical Council. *Confidentiality.* London: GMC; 2009.

16. Worthington R, Hays R. Responding to unprofessional behaviours. *Clin Teach.* 2012; **9**(2): 71–4.

17. Daniel AE, Burn RJ, Horarik S. Patients' complaints about medical practice. *Med J Aust.* 1999; **170**(12): 598–602.

18. Papadakis MA, Hodgson CS, Tehrani A, *et al.* Unprofessional behavior in medical school is associated with subsequent disciplinary action by a state medical board. *Acad Med.* 2004; **79**(3): 244–9.

19. General Medical Council. *Tomorrow's Doctors.* London: GMC; 2009. Available at: www.gmc-uk.org/education/undergraduate/tomorrows_doctors.asp (accessed 30 January 2013).

20. Ainsworth MA, Szauter KM. Medical student professionalism: are we developing the right behaviors? A comparison of professional lapses by students and physicians. *Acad Med.* 2006; **81**(10 Suppl.): S83–6.

21. Hodges BD, Ginsburg S, Cruess R, *et al.* Assessment of professionalism: recommendations from the Ottawa 2010 Conference. *Med Teach.* 2011; **33**(5): 354–63.

22. Wood L, Hassell A, Whitehouse A, *et al.* A literature review of multi-source feedback systems within and without healthcare services, leading to 10 tips for their successful design. *Med Teach.* 2006; **28**(7): e185–91.

23. Wilkinson T. Assessment of an individual's professionalism [symposium

presentation]. *15th Ottawa Conference: Assessment of Competence in Medicine and the Healthcare Professions*. 9–13 March 2012; Kuala Lumpur, Malaysia.

CHAPTER 3

Ethical analysis of professional issues in practice*

This chapter is where the main ethical analysis takes place, with the emphasis on applied ethics rather than ethical theory.

INTRODUCTION

In Part Two, the cases raise a range of issues that have relevance for medical educators, regulators and professional bodies, human resources and medical managers, doctors in training and, of course, patients. Some considerations arising from analysis of the cases are covered elsewhere in this book; for example, the relationship between ethics and professionalism is discussed in Chapter 2; educational matters are addressed in Chapters 2 and 4, regulatory and public policy issues are discussed in Chapters 2 and 5, and matters of patient safety are discussed at various points in the book. In this chapter the focus is on ethics, and among the topics covered are managerial and leadership issues relating to professional behaviours.

From looking at the questions inserted between the outline and the commentary of the cases in Part Two, the scope of ethical issues relating to unprofessional behaviours will become clear, and for logical reasons and reasons of convenience, the issues in this chapter are divided up as follows:

1. *Justice*: how does one go about balancing the need for fairness to be shown towards doctors and trainees against wider public or institutional interests, and are doctors and medical students ever 'a special case'?
2. *Responsibility*: who is ultimately accountable and to whom, and to what

---

* When reading this chapter, please cross-refer to Chapters 6 and 7 for practical illustrations of how these problems arise and how they might be addressed in particular cases.

extent are failings the result of poor management, poor leadership or poor educational policy (as opposed to the conduct and attitudes of the clinician)?

3. *Rights*: patients have rights, as well as other population groups, including health professionals and trainees. What is the best way of responding to professional problems that raise matters relating to human rights?

JUSTICE

Justice is not a single concept, and there are as many different ways of defining that which we call 'justice' as there are lawyers and philosophers. The type of justice that we are interested in here is societal justice, or justice as fairness, and not anything directly concerning governments or administrative categories of law. To put it another way, the question we seek to address at this juncture is that of balancing respect for the rights of the individual, who in our case is a doctor in training, against respecting the needs of society as a whole.

Before discussing *how* to achieve this balance, we need to consider the different parties. For a doctor or trainee in difficulty, perhaps facing a disciplinary panel, he or she is striving to protect a future career more than a professional reputation that is normally built up over time. Medical students and trainees invest money and effort in their training; they (and their families) often make sacrifices along the way so as to facilitate this investment. Even if somebody comes from an affluent family, for a medical student having to exit a course, possibly with no qualification at all, it is appropriate to take into consideration alternative careers and lost earnings had somebody chosen *not* to embark on medical training.

A trainee could have spent over 10 years in full-time education by the time he or she graduates. This level of commitment deserves some respect, as too does the fact that for somebody to reach that point and train in medicine at all, intelligence, application and a range of personal attributes, such as tenacity, patience and technical ability, are all needed in some measure in order to succeed. Fortunately, only a relatively small number of students or trainees lose focus and/or have to face disciplinary hearings, even though personal motivations for doing medicine may change with time.[1]

It could be argued that some of the difficulties that trainees face are self-inflicted, but it is unwise to be judgemental without knowing the facts surrounding an individual case. Some behaviours may be seen as a form of escape from pressures that go with the job, or they may simply be a sign of human frailty in coping with everyday stresses and strains, or of someone facing difficult personal circumstances. The authors know of medical students who find themselves in need of extra support resulting from a breakdown in personal relationships, from trying to protect a vulnerable member of the family, or from coping with other issues at home (including financial pressures or familial pressure to do medicine, when a student might have preferred to pursue a different career). Individual circumstances are as varied as life itself, but to take one example, we know of one student taking 6 years to complete the first 2 years of a 5-year programme on account of having time off for babies, time off for relationship difficulties, time off for illness, and having to resit examinations and repeat whole sections of the course.

To switch over and consider things from the societal perspective, the overriding public interest is usually patient safety, and several cases in Part Two have this high on the list of considerations. Even if a student or trainee is not directly responsible for the medical care of patients, he or she is an active member of the team that is responsible; whatever the reason, a trainee who is unsafe poses a hazard to the well-being of others, be they patients, peers or volunteers helping with clinical assessments and agreeing to be examined. The need to protect others from poorly performing doctors can have local, national or even international significance in that doctors sometimes move between countries, and there could be policy aspects to consider resulting from a scandal, such as changing the way that doctors are trained or regulated. Public interests are therefore quite varied, so it is wrong to think that medical training is a private or internal matter; ripples and waves that form after a problem case can be quite far-reaching.

The public has a strong interest in having a well-trained, safe workforce of health professionals; nobody wants to be treated by an incompetent doctor or have their loved ones suffer negligent care, and nobody wants a health service staffed by people who are poorly trained. For this reason the public often invests taxpayers' money in training and educating the healthcare workforce; the extent to which this happens varies between countries and locations. The actual arithmetic is of no concern to us here, although in the United Kingdom, many millions of pounds of public money change hands each year through medical schools paying compensation to hospitals and local service providers for help with teaching and training students.

Now, perhaps, we see how a balance has to be achieved between these different interests. There is no *direct* competition between individual and collective interests in terms of training doctors, because it is in everybody's interests to have a skilled, well-trained medical workforce. However, there is an element of *indirect* competition in that judgements have to be made between private and public interests, for instance, in allowing a medical student back onto a course or training programme, after a period of absence following a suspension.

Forcing somebody out of the medical profession is never the goal, even for a rigorous disciplinary committee, but making sure that an unsafe doctor does not go back to treating patients without first being investigated and then perhaps retrained, may well be the intention. As we have seen, investigating committees have a range of sanctions at their disposal, from suspension or exclusion from the programme at one end of the spectrum to arranging mentoring support or a student having to resit an exam at the other. While in rare cases somebody might have to consider pursuing an alternative career, public and private interests are usually better served by taking the necessary measures in order to try to rehabilitate a trainee facing difficulties.

Medical students and trainees have rights as citizens, as human beings and as proto-professionals, but having those rights does not put them above the law or put them into a category where they are somehow unassailable. This also applies to senior, experienced clinicians, whatever their status or reputation. Justice is not well served if medical professionals are seen as being too much of a special case. The medical profession has to *earn* public respect, and the individual doctor or trainee has to learn to do the same. Failing significantly to meet the requirements stipulated by regulatory bodies, medical schools or programme directors in terms of professional conduct means that he or she at some point has to face the consequences. Without checks and balances the process of training doctors could be chaotic, and as part of the business of protecting public interest, systems must be fair on those trainees who *do* perform to the required standard and who work hard and take good care of patients.

Panel members have to consider the facts of a case in front of them and do not have time to engage in philosophical debate about the rights and wrongs of public policy. However, it is good to consider these issues from time to time, as they have significance for the whole enterprise of training health professionals. Due process matters to everyone, including the person subject to a formal disciplinary inquiry as well as the wider public. Overall, 'justice as fairness' is probably the best motto to adopt in this regard, as it allows time and space for the interests of society to be weighed against the rights of the individual.[2]

RESPONSIBILITY

Although responsibility and rights go hand in hand, we choose to address them here as separate issues, partly for convenience of organisation and partly because the focus now is on management and leadership more than the responsibility and obligations of individuals. Disciplinary hearings sometimes highlight shortcomings in systems, procedures and management structure, bringing to the surface issues that might hitherto have been neglected. For instance, this could happen with a new school where systems have not been properly tested, or in an established programme where systems have not been brought up to date to incorporate new professional standards or changes in the law. Faculty deans and heads of school not only have to ensure that appropriate committee structures are in place and that suitable members of staff are first identified and then appropriately trained, but they must also make sure that senior faculty are aware of new standards or changes in the law so that everything is 'fit for purpose'. For a new medical school it may only be weeks or months into a programme before problems arise with student behaviours, and it is not fair on those individuals to be subjected to poorly evolved systems or be assessed by untrained staff. These matters have to be addressed in a timely fashion in order to be fair to everyone involved, both individually and collectively.

One potential hazard, discussed in Part Two, is where a school committee reaches a decision on a professionalism issue but the decision is subsequently overturned on appeal – for example, where the parent organisation (a university or teaching hospital) is working to a different set of standards from the school. If a trainee is 'let off the hook' by an appeals committee because its members are unfamiliar with risk assessment from the point of view of the general public and the legal responsibilities that go hand in hand with running a medical training programme, then patients may be being put at risk. A medical degree is not just a programme of education, where lack of maturity or lack or experience might be condoned in the early years; medicine is a professional training that directly and indirectly involves members of the public. In that schools are bringing in opportunities for clinical experience into what used to be considered preclinical years, this gives the matter added poignancy.[3]

When assessing professional behaviour, a question that needs asking is 'who ultimately is accountable to whom?' As suggested at the beginning of this chapter, and as discussed further in Part Two, the extent to which individual failings are the result of poor management, poor leadership or poor educational policy needs proper evaluation. It is not fair, for instance, if a trainee is sanctioned because he or she happened to be caught in the crossfire between two 'warring' senior members of staff, or if internal protocols have not been properly thought through. Probity and professionalism need to be displayed by all parties to the enterprise of training doctors; educators are just as accountable, if not more so, than those who are being educated. It is no good having one standard for students and another for clinical teachers, who could be seen exhibiting standards of professional conduct that would not be tolerated from a student. This would be unjust, and unethical, but it is a real problem and one that is not that easy to address, as it goes right to the heart of the way in which medicine in practised. Role modelling is a part of the general strategy for educating doctors, but not all influences to which a doctor will be exposed are necessarily going to be positive.[4,5]

RIGHTS

People are sometimes afraid of rights, and this fear may stem from apprehension about saying the wrong thing and causing offence. At other times the question of rights is not the real issue and may perhaps be a smokescreen that is being created to divert attention away from some other issue. The difficulty is knowing 'which is which' and when it is appropriate to speak out. If sexism, for instance, is rife in the workplace it is not merely right and proper to bring it up, it is a moral duty. Patterns of behaviour can go unchallenged for long periods of time unless someone speaks out, but we recognise that it can be very difficult, especially for somebody junior when it means challenging the authority of someone in a senior position. It takes courage to speak out, and, regrettably, careers have been blighted as a result of having stood up for the rights of others, and there are few (if any) incentives for someone to speak out and challenge unprofessional conduct.

In the cases presented in Part Two of this book, rights are never the primary focus; it is more often the case that rights issues are brought up because of some other problem or behaviour; nonetheless, rights often forms the subtext behind a case in terms of the way in which a case pans out. For instance, mental health problems are not uncommon among medical students, and while mental health rights may not be explicitly addressed, attitudes towards mental health may be part of the reason why a student or trainee chooses to keep something hidden, or part of the reason why a committee decides to act in a certain way (e.g. by calling for a psychiatric opinion before coming to a conclusion about possible disciplinary action).

To take another example, if a medical student or junior doctor reveals bullying in the workplace, this could be brushed aside and treated as an irrelevance, perhaps in order to protect a senior colleague. Such a response would not be ethically appropriate and the matter should be investigated, regardless of seniority or the identity of the alleged perpetrator. In addition, if several people make similar allegations then it is more likely that someone in authority will sit up and take note. An example where this could apply could be the ritual humiliation of medical students by senior clinicians in front of peers, patients and professionals. Once it was perhaps thought of as a 'rite of passage' and something that 'goes with the territory of learning to be a doctor', but such behaviour is ethically indefensible; those who continue to behave in that way are being unprofessional and disrespectful of the rights of the individual and should expect to be censored. Students have rights too, however junior they are within the medical hierarchy.[6,7]

Racial and ethnic slurs can be especially difficult to deal with, and, regrettably, incidents sometimes arise in which a trainee belonging to an ethnic minority alleges racism on the part of a colleague in order to deflect attention away from a personal weakness or failing, such as an emotional inability to cope with some forms of pressure. This could happen at any point in someone's career; as with sexism or bullying allegations, it is a question of seeking to identify when and if there is a real issue of racial intolerance, and when and if it is being used as a smokescreen. Dealing with issues such as these is never easy, and processes of investigation can take up a great deal of staff time and energy. However, that may be unavoidable, and it would be wrong simply to ignore such allegations, since it may lead to a greater harm, with others falling victim to the same thing later on. Even in a classroom setting it can be challenging raising issues around race and ethnicity; sometimes students or trainees are simply not willing to discuss this topic in front of their peers.

If a rights problem does exist and needs dealing with, it is almost always better for the individual affected to seek out an experienced member of staff or to raise the issue with a personal or clinical tutor. If any student or trainee falls victim to bullying, victimisation or sexual innuendo, it can be more than just demoralising; it can harm his or her mental and physical health, and in turn it can hold back his or her career and affect other members of the student or trainee's family. In other words, a problem that goes unaddressed is transferred from the person displaying the inappropriate behaviour on to someone in a weaker position who is meant to 'bottle it up' and just stay silent. It is a sad day when a teacher hears of such a case, knowing that a talented, capable individual is facing this type of challenge. That said, unless someone speaks out then those in authority are unaware or else unable to act. Therefore, providing proof is important, and for the person seeking to make a complaint, it would be a good first step to find someone who is having a similar experience or someone who witnessed the problem behaviour in question. It is then more likely that a senior tutor or manager will take the matter up, inform someone in authority (such as a head of school or human resources personnel) and take the appropriate action.

The following cases in Part Two specifically involve rights issues:

- Case 13: human rights (in general)
- Case 26: population rights
- Case 10: racial discrimination
- Case 7: gender issues and sexual discrimination
- Cases 4, 15, 17 and 24: mental health
- Cases 12 and 9: bullying
- Cases 14 and 19: disability rights
- Cases 27 and 28: liberty rights.

Patient rights are also an important factor, and these are not ignored when we analyse the cases in Part Two. However, not all responsibility falls on the healthcare practitioner. Patients have responsibilities too, such as to communicate fairly with clinicians, not to physically or verbally abuse them, and to play a part in arriving at a shared decision as part of the process of consent. Clinician and patient need to negotiate a course of action that respects patient values and preferences, recognises any clinical limitations that might exist and recognises the rights of the clinician to express a professional opinion (while stopping short of being too coercive).

To explore these matters further we would like to focus on two topics from the list given: (1) matters of gender and sexualised behaviour and (2) problems relating to mental health and disability.

Gender and sexualised behaviour

While problems relating to gender discrimination may have improved as a result of efforts to raise standards of professionalism in the workplace and the introduction of human rights legislation,[8,9] anecdotal evidence suggests that this form of discrimination remains a problem. Furthermore, it may not necessarily be perpetrated by someone in a position of power; for instance, the authors know of a case involving a second-year international medical student who found it difficult reading signals from members of the opposite sex and who thought that friendly gestures (such as touching an arm) were expressions of sexual interest. He complained that a lab technician and some female students were behaving inappropriately; however, when challenged about these complaints and asked to substantiate the allegation he tried to deflect attention, accusing a respected member of staff of displaying racial discrimination towards *him*. In another instance, a female American trainee saw no problem in mimicking some of her male colleagues and making sexualised comments. The scenario outlined in Case 7 (*see* Part Two) was, for various reasons, not easy for senior faculty to deal with and find a satisfactory solution to the problem. Such cases are never easy, but to ignore them would, in our view, be a greater wrong.

When going about the task of investigating it is worth bearing in mind the risk that a case may be undermined by poor systems and procedures; even strong cases can be overturned on appeal if the right person did not take the right course of action at the right time. This applies equally to complaints against medical students as it does to complaints against doctors in training; in the case of the latter, human resources and employment law are necessarily part of the mix, as well as published professional standards and in-house policies and procedures. Managers of medical schools and training programmes need to be sure not only that they have good processes and procedures in place but also that these systems meet current legal standards and are generally fit for purpose.

More commonly, it is the case that a clinician might be tempted to abuse his power (yes, it does tend to be men that display this type of behaviour) – for example, making repeated innuendos about 'attractive' junior female members of staff, or commenting on physical characteristics of an anaesthetised patient in such a way as to cause offence to members of the team. Sexualised behaviour does not have to involve physical contact in order for it to be unprofessional, inappropriate and/or in breach of someone's rights.

However, proving any form of discrimination can be difficult, and this is no less the case when it comes to gender issues. Paradoxically, where a case involves sexual intercourse – for instance, a clinician having an inappropriate relationship with a junior colleague or with a patient in his or her care – it may be easier to deal with. It is likely that in such a case the matter would be escalated and reach the point either where a doctor or trainee is suspended from work or where a case is reported to the regulator for formal investigation. That incidents involving intimate relations take place from time to time is a matter of record,[10] and they come to public attention by reason of the gravity of the offending behaviour. However, it is the subtle cases that are often harder to deal with – for example, in the absence of sufficiently robust evidence, either because the person wronged does not want to come forward and formalise a complaint or because the person who is being investigated puts on a good front and the panel does not know whose account to believe.

Mental health and disability concerns

Doctors are at risk of suffering mental health problems no less than other sectors of the population; in fact, they may be more prone to experiencing difficulty with depression, which can be hard for anyone to handle, including doctors, and particularly during training (e.g. when decisions have to be made about if or when to disclose something that could hinder future careers and where 'not to disclose' could be dishonest and unprofessional). Medical schools are generally keen to detect possible psychiatric problems as early as possible so as to be able to offer appropriate help and support. Such problems can manifest through a range of different behaviours, including unexplained absences and/or unexpectedly poor performance in exams, both of which can lead to a student being called before a committee to explain what is happening. The common expectation is perhaps that a doctor should be used to coping with difficult situations, and while this may be true when it applies to others, doctors and trainees are not immune to having their own personal problems and stresses – for example, arising from relationship difficulties, disturbed sleep, eating disorders, obsessive–compulsive behaviours, or simply juggling multiple responsibilities, perhaps with dependants at home and significant demands being placed on someone's capacity to work and/or study.[11-13]

Doctors in training need help and support during difficult times, and if they do not receive it, cracks may begin to appear in terms of their professional behaviours and how they present to others (including patients). Several cases in Part Two touch on a problem sometimes faced by medical educators and others in positions of responsibility: when is it appropriate to offer support and encouragement, and when is it necessary to act in the public interest and remove somebody from situations where harm could be caused to others? Often as not, if pressures are building it does the trainee a favour by temporarily removing them from the workplace in order to give external matters a chance to be sorted, and thus possibly preventing harm from being caused to patients and colleagues, as well as further career difficulties arising from problems that remain unresolved.

Rehabilitation is often the best and most appropriate course of action to take – for example, by a clinical tutor or supervisor wishing to take appropriate supportive action without neglecting the public duty to protect others. This is especially the case when it comes to addictive behaviours, which are not uncommon among medical professionals (several cases in Part Two deal with drug-related difficulties). For instance, in the case of alcohol, a doctor found to be driving while over the legal limit could face immediate suspension from work, even before his or her case has time to be investigated. The next step could be compulsory attendance at specialist clinics for dealing with addictive behaviours, and while this curtails the autonomy of the doctor or trainee it is probably the lesser harm, from the point of view of both public protection and safeguarding future medical careers (and the public investment that goes into the provision of training).[14,15]

In law, mental health is classified as a form of disability.[16] This is accurate and meaningful in that mental health problems can significantly hinder somebody's life chances – for instance, regarding employment, personal relations and other matters of health. However, the breadth of this definition is not without implication for a professional and it may serve to hinder somebody from coming forward and seeking psychiatric help, especially in that the fact of the matter is likely to become a permanent part of someone's medical record. That said, undiagnosed or untreated problems can obstruct the delivery of good-quality, safe care to patients, and it thus becomes a matter of ethical as well as clinical judgement to determine which course of action is most appropriate, carrying with it the least risk of harm – for example, to treat, to not treat but simply monitor, to take time off sick and/or to notify appropriate 'others'.

In short, a trainee whose problem is not being treated effectively is a risk to him- or herself regarding general health and well-being, as well as posing a potential risk to others such as patients, peers and colleagues, and if a problem grows then people in positions of seniority may have to become involved. With doctors in difficulty, investigating panels are likely to be aware of the possibility of an underlying mental health problem being the root cause of unprofessional conduct, and while some trainees will have difficulties in managing their condition, which is first a health problem and second a professional problem, the disability aspects of mental health need further consideration.

There is a positive side to this classification, such as entitlements to support in the workplace, as well as sickness and other state benefits, and for the medical school or trainee, it should be in the best interests of the individual to come clean and explain difficulties associated with having a disability so that help can be offered and suitable accommodations can be made. Schools and employers are bound by law to respect the rights of individuals with a disability, including those with mental health concerns.[11] However, there is still the question of stigma that needs to be addressed, which is not something that can easily be done through legislation or issuing professional guidance.[17] It is more a matter of public awareness, tolerance and understanding, as well as something with which an individual may simply have to come to terms.

REFERENCES

1. Worthington R, Obhrai M. Personal and professional values: responses from a questionnaire survey of Foundation year one doctors [presentation]. *Midlands NHS Deanery Conference.* 19 May 2011; Birmingham, UK.
2. Sen A. *The Idea of Justice.* Cambridge, MA: Belknap Press; 2011.
3. Yardley S, Littlewood S, Margolis SA, *et al.* What has changed in the evidence for early experience? Update of a BEME systematic review. *Med Teach.* 2010; **32**(9): 740–6.
4. Ainsworth MA, Szauter KM. Medical student professionalism: are we developing the right behaviors? A comparison of professional lapses by students and physicians. *Acad Med.* 2006; **81**(10 Suppl.): S83–6.
5. Cruess SR, Cruess RL, Steinert Y. Role modelling: making the most of a powerful teaching strategy. *BMJ.* 2008; **336**(7646): 718–21.
6. Council of Heads of Medical School; British Medical Association students. *Medical School Charter.* London: British Medical Association; 2006. Available at: www.currexec. mvm.ed.ac.uk/docs/open/MedicalSchoolCharter.pdf (accessed 7 January 2013).
7. Crutcher RA, Szafran O, Woloschuk W, *et al.* Family medicine graduates' perceptions of intimidation, harassment, and discrimination during residency training. *BMC Med Educ.* 2011; **11**: 88. Available at: www.biomedcentral.com/content/pdf/1472-6920-11-88.pdf (accessed 17 January 2013).
8. Human Rights Act 1998. Available at: www.legislation.gov.uk/ukpga/1998/42/contents (accessed 17 January 2013).
9. Equality Act 2010. Available at: www.legislation.gov.uk/ukpga/2010/15/contents (accessed 8 May 2013).
10. General Medical Council. *Decisions.* Available at: www.gmc-uk.org/concerns/hearings _and_decisions/fitness_to_practise_decisions.asp (accessed 8 May 2013).

11. Tyssen R, Vaglum P. Mental health problems among young doctors: an updated review of prospective studies. *Harv Rev Psychiatry*. 2002; **10**(3): 154–65.

12. Chew-Graham CA, Rogers A, Yassin N. I wouldn't want it on my CV or their records: medical students' experiences of help-seeking for mental health problems. *Med Educ*. 2003; **37**(10): 873–80.

13. Grässel E, Lampen-Imkamp S, Lehrl S, *et al*. Screening of emotional and somatic complaints in undergraduate medical students: a longitudinal study [German]. *Psychiatr Prax*. 2013; **40**(1): 30–5. Available at: www.ncbi.nlm.nih.gov/pubmed/23319281 (accessed 17 January 2013).

14. Jackson AH, Alford DP, Dubé CE, *et al*. Internal medicine residency training for unhealthy alcohol and other drug use: recommendations for curriculum design. *Med Educ*. 2010; **10**: 22. Available at: www.biomedcentral.com/content/pdf/1472-6920-10-22.pdf (accessed 17 January 2013).

15. Grotmol KS, Vaglum P, Ekeberg O, *et al*. Alcohol expectancy and hazardous drinking: a 6-year longitudinal and nationwide study of medical doctors. *Eur Addict Res*. 2010; **16**(1): 17–22. Available at: http://content.karger.com/ProdukteDB/produkte. asp?Aktion=ShowPDF&ArtikelNr=000253860&Ausgabe=253652&ProduktNr=224 233&filename=000253860.pdf (accessed 17 January 2013).

16. Disability Discrimination Act 1995 [updated 2005]. Available at: www.legislation. gov.uk/ukpga/1995/50/contents (accessed 19 January 2013).

17. Corrigan P. How stigma interferes with mental health care. *Am Psychol*. 2004; **59**(7): 614–25.

CHAPTER 4

International trends in medical education: professionalism in context

In this chapter we talk about social and historical aspects to professionalism, as well as shifting views and influences on how professionalism comes to be understood by the professions and by society as a whole. We also consider issues relating to selection into medical programmes and some difficulties that arise when professionals cross national borders.

INTRODUCTION

It is perhaps too obvious to state that the nature of professionalism in healthcare has evolved over recent times. In many respects, the original tenets of the Hippocratic oath have not changed, and after surviving for over 2000 years they continue to have meaning, in spite of major changes that have taken place in medicine. Medicine has evolved from near-religious caring and comforting of the ill, with little prospect of cure, giving way to a highly scientific and rational approach to preventing and fighting disease, with high expectations of achieving good outcomes. However, professionalism has changed over time, and it will continue to change in the way it is defined, demonstrated and measured. The world is now a more cosmopolitan and connected place, with nations being made up of a healthy mix of ethnic, religious and cultural groups in both the population and the healthcare workforce, albeit with differing degrees of harmony.

This chapter focuses on recent changes, illustrating contemporary views through consideration of a series of cases that authors have encountered in their recent careers as clinicians, teachers, researchers and/or education managers. The cases below may look superficially similar, but each took place at a different time and in a different country.

Consider the following:

Case A: 1980s, Australia – a mid-level medical student at a well-known medical school drove home from a medical student society party one Saturday night after consuming alcohol, hit a tree after trying to take a corner at speed, and was given a breathalyser test by the police. The result was positive, and a higher than permitted blood alcohol level was confirmed as being three times the legal limit on a blood test. Luckily, no one was injured in the accident. A few weeks later the student pleaded guilty to a charge of driving under the influence (rather than driving dangerously), and his driving licence was suspended for 6 months. The case was reported in the local newspaper, including mention of the fact that he was a 'university student'. The medical school took no action, regarding this as being an essentially private matter. His friends thought he was lucky, and he gained a kind of respect for having 'beaten the system'. He went on to successfully complete the course and is now a respected senior clinician.

Case B: 1990s, United States – a senior medical student at a prestigious medical school drove home from a party one Saturday night after consuming alcohol; he was noticed by police to be driving erratically and was pulled over and given a breathalyser test. He returned a higher than permitted blood alcohol level, which was confirmed on a blood test. A few weeks later the student pleaded guilty to driving under the influence of alcohol; he was penalised by suspension of his driving licence for a period of 6 months. This conviction was reported in the local newspaper, including his connection to the prestigious school. The school leaders referred him to a disciplinary panel on a charge of 'bringing the university into disrepute'. He was found 'guilty', and he was expelled from the school without being able to return to complete the course.

Case C: 2000s, United Kingdom – a senior medical student at one of the new medical schools drove home from a party one Saturday night after consuming alcohol. He was noticed by police to be driving too fast; he was stopped and given a breathalyser test, which showed a higher than permitted blood alcohol level and this was confirmed on a blood test. A few weeks later he pleaded guilty in court and his licence was suspended for a period of 6 months. The medical school referred him to the Fitness to Practise Committee. As a condition of staying on the course he was referred for psychiatric assessment with regard to possible alcohol dependence; he was required not to offend again but faced no actual penalty. He successfully completed the course and is currently nearing completion of his specialty training.

Case D: 2010s, Australia – a senior medical student at a well-known medical school drove home from a party one Saturday night after consuming alcohol. Although driving normally, he was pulled over at a police random breath testing unit and found to have a higher than permitted blood alcohol reading. This was confirmed on a blood test as being just over the legal limit. A few weeks later he pleaded guilty in court and his driving licence was suspended for a period of 6 months. The medical school referred him to the Fitness to Practise Committee. As a condition of staying on the course he was referred for psychiatric assessment of possible alcohol dependence and was required not to offend again. He was also notified to the Australian Health Practitioner Regulation Agency as a potential health risk to patients. This means that if he does not re-offend and then graduates, he will be subject to a formal health assessment prior to commencing work. Furthermore, although his career will be unimpeded if he does not reoffend, his offence as a student will be permanently attached to his professional registration record.

These cases highlight several interesting and important issues. First, there are differences between countries and in how common issues of possible unprofessionalism are regarded by society and managed by regulators. Tolerance of certain behaviours varies with time, and while attitudes to alcohol in Australia could be seen as more relaxed than they are in the United States, there may be other elements at play. For instance, one could compare original colonising populations of mostly Irish convicts with deeply religious pilgrims and not be too surprised at the differences in culture. Furthermore, in the United Kingdom as in other Western nations, many medical students are now Islamic, and according to the tenets of the Islamic faith, alcohol is simply forbidden. This extends to the point where although alcohol might be available at extra cost, medical student parties no longer provide alcohol as a matter of routine. As a corollary to this, the use of drugs other than alcohol (e.g. 'party drugs', such as nitrous oxide canisters) may be popular as an alternative to alcohol and other types of stimulant.

Second, times change, and looking at the two Australian cases, separated by 30 years, it is clear that attitudes to medical students who drink too much alcohol have changed substantially. What was once regarded as a 'private and personal matter', 'high spirits', 'part of growing up' and something 'relatively harmless' is now regarded as a professionalism issue and viewed as a likely indicator of a recurring problem with alcohol that could ultimately affect patient safety.

Third, as a result of these changes, processes for managing cases of professionals with alcohol problems have similarly had to evolve. There are now relevant regulations, formal referral structures and processes, as well as disciplinary and remedial pathways. Furthermore, the initially firm disciplinary approach seen in the US case is now most likely to be replaced, or at least augmented, by alternative processes that are health focused and which offer remediation.

WHY HAS PROFESSIONALISM ASSUMED INCREASED IMPORTANCE?

The nature of healthcare is changing from an individual to a system pursuit. While romantic tales remain, with heroic efforts by amazing individuals (doctors usually get the credit), modern healthcare is increasingly delivered by teams of people with complementary skills that combine to produce better health outcomes. Common examples include high-acuity areas such as emergency rooms, operating theatres and intensive care units, where every staff member has a specific role that requires the application of specific knowledge and skills, the following of clinical protocols and to be supported by evidence-based guidelines. Patient survival and quality of life depend more on teams doing their job well than on one individual doing something heroic.

Similarly, much of the success in primary care requires teams of people to help maintain health, prevent illness, diagnose early and manage appropriately. This includes coordinating care across several different specialties and services, particularly those that target chronic diseases. These tasks require more than medical practitioners, who not so long ago had to provide primary care almost single-handedly. Other health professionals now perform tasks such as vaccination monitoring and chronic disease management, with the general practitioners acting more as a consultant to the team, contributing expertise in complex diagnostic cases and making managerial decisions. Teamwork is not just about people in the same profession working together; it is people working together across the professions, which is where interprofessional education and assessment come into play. Real teamwork is better developed when real teams work in the real world (or with high-fidelity simulations).[1]

One possible reason for this shift is that healthcare has become more

complex and technological, making it difficult for an individual in a single profession to provide all aspects of care required for treating patients. As a result,
the scope of expertise for individuals has narrowed, so that healthcare requires
access to several different kinds of expertise and, hence, several different individuals (and professions). The number of recognised specialties continues to
grow, although generalism remains important to provide a view across nar-
rower specialties.

Another reason is that much more is known about the issues affecting the
safety and quality of healthcare.[2,3] A surprisingly (and alarmingly) high proportion of adverse events and outcomes appear to be ascribed, at least in part,
to errors made by individuals who are acting alone, tired from long working
hours, unwell or affected by alcohol or other drugs. All of these factors are
regarded as preventable, and the failure of an organisation to address these
factors could ultimately lead to criminal charges being brought.[4] For example,
medication dosages must be checked by a second person, 'safe' work hours
have been defined in some jurisdictions[5] and there are robust procedures for
addressing health and drug-related problems.

GENERATIONAL CHANGE

Generational change is a more recently described phenomenon that captures
the concept of societal changes in attitudes, beliefs and behaviours that occur
over time, which roughly correlate with certain age groups. Although there
is more likely to be a gradual evolution over time, it is convenient to think
of generalised characteristics of groups of people. This used to be described
according to major political, economic or industrial developments, relating to
'the Victorian era', 'the Great Depression' or a period relating to major wars.
We now tend to think of attributes of 'a generation', rather than 'an era'. This
implies that societal change has hastened or perhaps been more studied from
about the mid-twentieth century onwards, commencing with the baby-boomer
or post-World War II generation.

While most families are microcosms demonstrating ways in which inter-
generational differences are played out, the phenomenon has interesting
implications for healthcare. A substantial proportion of current health workers,
particularly at senior and leadership levels, are baby boomers, who typically
work long hours, remain loyal to organisations (including employers) and
believe in providing after-hours care as part of 24-hour, 7-day-a-week professional responsibility. This comes at the expense of personal lifestyle options,
and people have been happy to wait their turn for seniority-related leadership
opportunities to come along.

The junior members of health professions provide the sharpest contrast.

People born in the 1980s and 1990s, known as 'Generation Y' or 'Millennials', for instance, want to work defined hours and 'have a life'. They are a larger group than 'Generation X', born between 1965 and 1980, and they make up a growing body of the workforce.[6] Millennials are happy to switch organisations (e.g. banks, telephone companies and probably employers) in search of better deals, and, more to the point, they are inclined to be ambitious in wanting leadership as soon as possible, perhaps emulating role models such as young information technology gurus who become billionaires by early adulthood.[7] They are extraordinarily connected via contemporary information technology, and, worryingly for educators, they may not be well suited to more traditional medical school teaching models. From a policy perspective, with baby boomers (born between 1945 and 1965) leaving the workforce during the next 10 years, interesting questions arise about what happens when these 'stable, loyal, dutiful workers' move on and retire.

While we stress that these generalisations do not describe all people within the categories, amid these characteristics, changes are emerging in relation to certain aspects of professionalism. For instance, junior health professionals are more likely to have poor on-time attendance, place unwise or inappropriate information on social media sites,[8,9] argue the 'fine print' of regulations, and bring in barristers to contest failed examination decisions. Where more senior

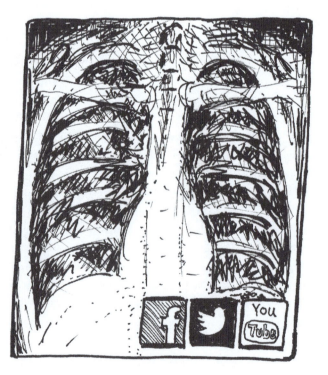

workers might have problems with alcohol and prescription drugs (narcotics and sedatives), younger workers might be having problems with 'party drugs' (e.g. *see* Cases 1, 3 and 27 in Part Two).

OTHER SOCIETAL CHANGES

While it is convenient to think about generational changes as influencing how society works, changes are occurring that affect people of any and all ages. Information technology is not the preserve of the young, but rather it is something that has been developing for some time. Therefore, it is the case that we live in an era of rapid communication with information that is easily accessible. Members of the public tend to want to know more about everything and to seek information that will help them to make the choices that suit them best. As a result, public awareness of all types of information is often high, and patients might arrive at a consultation after having first conducted an internet search. While professionals can criticise search engines that are not underpinned by rigorous assessment and strength of evidence, patients feel (and often are) better informed about their health now than in the past.

Another broad characteristic that may result from increased public awareness is that we are moving away from an era of patient (and learner) 'centredness' and towards one of 'partnership'. Groups as well as individuals have views on what might be expected or achieved, and it is increasingly difficult for health professionals to achieve better health outcomes without overt engagement from members of 'society'.[10] Patients will no longer just do what the doctor says; instead, they want acknowledgement of who they are and to be part of the solution for their problems. For example, a commonly used and effective screening tool for bowel cancer is regular faecal occult blood testing. However, uptake rates tend to be higher when people do this as part of a community-based campaign rather than simply when a doctor recommends it.[11] Many public health campaigns are often based on community group action, such as service clubs, acting in partnership with professional organisations.

Another example is health workforce planning. Not very long ago, universities would decide how many health professionals to train based on their own strategic plans, which usually had little relationship to community need, whereas governments now prefer to 'commission' the required number of graduates.[12] An important outcome of this increased communication and community engagement is that there is now a more shared view on what professionalism may or may not be. Just as information about health, disease and illness is more detailed and more accessible, so too is information about breaches in professionalism. Almost everybody has heard about the worst (highly publicised) cases of poor performance and doctors behaving badly, which we discuss in the next chapter, each of which led to major public inquiries.[13-16] This had the effect of 'demonising' some institutions and individuals, focusing on very poor rather than sound or aspirational models of professionalism. Nonetheless, it has arguably resulted in a greater public awareness both of the importance of professionalism and of situations where professionalism was found seriously wanting.

GLOBALISATION OF MEDICAL EDUCATION

With modern communications technology enabling rapid transmission of information around the world, internet access is now available in most countries, and there may be almost as many mobile phones as there are people on the planet. Many of these phones have movie cameras, allowing the immediate recording and dissemination of news events. In July 2005 one of the authors (RH) watched live the aftermath of the bombing of buses and trains in London from a time zone 10 hours ahead, before a colleague at a UK university, who happened to be on a 'live' email exchange, even knew that it was happening. This is now no longer unusual, because with Twitter accounts, for example, people often hear about events as they are actually happening, sometimes even before the police or media. The 'Arab Spring' of 2011–12 saw regime change come about after being managed by social media, with information that was spread rapidly within and across national boundaries.

Healthcare and health professional education are now also global enterprises. Some nations deliberately aim to be 'health hubs' or 'health education hubs', developing excellent facilities in order to attract patients from other nations. In addition, university health professional programmes attracting international students generate a form of 'export commodity' post graduation. This is helped by the regional accreditation of programmes that increases the portability of medical qualifications and facilitates the migration of medical graduates to where the employment opportunities lie.

There is a move towards an international accreditation approach, affording mutual recognition by regional accreditation agencies that follow international guidelines, which the World Federation for Medical Education (WFME) is currently promoting.[17] While local assessments, including licensing examinations, are often required before international graduates can practise in another jurisdiction, in some respects, international recognition of basic medical qualifications is now less of a barrier to migration than obtaining the right visa. This globalisation of medical education brings into focus the differences in curricula that become particularly evident when making international comparisons. More traditional curricula, including those in both developed and developing nations, are often strong on biomedical science but weak on behavioural and social science, ethics and professionalism. As we saw in Chapter 2, these curriculum areas are often not well assessed, if they are addressed at all.

WFME Basic Medical Education Standards require these topics to be covered, but even schools with a WFME 'stamp of approval' show considerable variation in the content of their curricula. Hence, it is possible for an international medical graduate to gain a licence in one jurisdiction, featuring strong biomedical science and clinical skills that meet internationally agreed standards, but have little or no training in ethics, professionalism or healthcare organisation. In consequence, international medical graduates tend to be over-represented in relation to their numbers in matters such as these when brought to the attention of local regulatory authorities.

CULTURAL ISSUES

An often-stated reason for the over-representation of international medical graduates in professionalism concerns is when there is a difference in culture between the nation of origin and the nation of practice. In most respects, professional roles and responsibilities are similar in all healthcare settings – doctors are always in a position of trust, are tacitly permitted to ask personal questions and conduct sensitive examinations, and are expected to be non-judgemental about cultural preferences in healthcare. However, a few standout issues of difference are specific to certain cultures.

One example is alleged sexism within the more traditional, paternalistic cultures, whereby doctor–patient interactions would either be gender matched or conducted in the presence of a chaperone. This can pose a challenge within Western society, where healthcare is delivered by women as much as (or even more than) men, and in liberal Western society it is no longer thought necessary, appropriate or, for that matter, feasible to provide chaperones for anything other than intimate examinations (if requested). For doctors raised under less liberal social systems, this can be challenging, especially during training, when Western norms and expectations are still unfamiliar, which can easily go on and lead to misunderstandings (e.g. *see* Case 12 in Part Two).

Another example is concern over forms of headwear that reduce people's ability to identify a healthcare professional and read their non-verbal signals, and patients may feel uncomfortable if they are unable to see the doctor's face. Situations such as these give rise to communication barriers; nonetheless, it may not be right simply to ban headwear that is worn for reasons of strong personal conviction. Solutions may only be found after having a meaningful and open debate.

Another cultural problem is to do with expectations of certain forms of behaviour associated with strongly hierarchical social structures. Since modern healthcare is increasingly about teamwork and mutual responsibility, natural deference to seniority and hierarchy can make it difficult for doctors to adapt to the modern environment. In addition, senior doctors could feel affronted if questioned by a junior colleague, but it could be simply that they are speaking out in order to try to prevent an error.

Finally, patients may not feel comfortable asking questions about healthcare options if that type of behaviour is not the social or cultural norm to which they are accustomed. Therefore, they may not want to take part fully in making informed decisions. It is primarily a case of forming personal judgements about when to respect cultural traditions and when something needs to be challenged. However, while professional standards in the host country have to be respected, doctors cannot put themselves outside the law, making social judgements in professional situations. The issues that we describe are sensitive and can apply to people of any nationality, race, religion or creed, and it is important to remember that forming judgements should not lead to unreasonable discriminatory actions.

NATIONAL JURISDICTIONAL ISSUES

Different nations have different political structures and legal systems, to a point where very similar issues may be managed differently, even if the legal systems are broadly similar, as in the countries covered by this book. Laws change over time in response to societal changes, albeit slowly, and in the long run, laws tend to reflect local societal norms. From the perspective of the health professions, the local legal system and nation in which the professional works are important factors, as can be seen in these examples.

The first concerns the personal use of cannabis by a doctor. While not condoned anywhere, in some jurisdictions this could lead to a criminal conviction with consequences extending beyond the end of a career, while in others the key issue is merely whether or not the doctor is free of drugs 'during work hours'. The second example is euthanasia and physician-assisted suicide, which is legal under certain circumstances in some nations but career-ending and a criminal offence in others. A third example is an international medical student from a socially conservative country who is studying in a modern, developed country in which locally acceptable student behaviours would be viewed as 'immoral' back at home. If the trainee decides to join in, they risk sanction if and when they return home, or if they criticise their peers and, worse still, their patients, they risk local sanction for poor professionalism and/or social isolation.

Another contemporary and interesting issue concerns the position of health professionals who work in more than one nation; this appears to be increasingly common in our connected, 'shrinking' world. There are international agencies that place health professionals for periods of time in mostly developing nations, particularly for humanitarian purposes. Other health professionals might take this simply as an opportunity to earn more money. For example, medical practitioners from Europe can earn high incomes for weekend locum positions in the United Kingdom (similarly, with New Zealand doctors working in Australia). These arrangements can be risky to patients as well as to doctors, in both mainstream and locum roles, because tiredness can increase the risk of medical error. Furthermore, it is difficult for health practitioners to be able to conform to expected standards of professionalism in more than one health and legal system. It is likely that sound professionalism is sufficiently similar for most doctors to be able to adapt and manage. However, this means being aware of the need to adapt in each different location and taking care to observe local, cultural, religious and perhaps political norms.

More complex, perhaps, is how poor professionalism in one nation is managed when a health professional moves across national borders. This used to mean restarting careers with a clean sheet, particularly if the professional did not declare his or her history of problems in other jurisdictions, as happened in one notable Australian example.[14] Most medical councils and boards now share information and have made non-declaration of problems in other jurisdictions a very serious breach that could be sufficient as to be able to prevent registration.

SELECTING FOR PROFESSIONALISM

One almost perennial problem affecting medical education is finding ways to reduce serious professional problems and prevent them from occurring through improved processes of selection. The question is most relevant to medicine because that is where the demand outstrips the places that are available, and there is evidence that students with professional problems are well represented in medical board disciplinary matters in later years.[18]

Many medical schools assess personal as well as academic qualities, but the instruments and measures used are imprecise. Testimonials are probably poor predictors, and 'morality' questions in aptitude tests are as yet unproven. Even interviews that are high on face validity appear not to reduce by much the small numbers of students with personal problems who go on to cause professional concerns. The recent multiple mini-interview method shows promising predictive validity, but so far this has been used mostly at postgraduate specialist entry level.[19]

There are different challenges for selection processes for school-leavers (about 18 years of age) compared with entrants with prior degrees who have more life experience. There is still much to be done to improve understanding of the issues before selection processes can be relied on to improve the professionalism of medical graduates. It is unlikely that selection methods alone will stop or prevent poor professionalism, but when combined with a range of assessment tools and early identification and remediation strategies, together they might be able to reduce the number and/or severity of problems when they arise.

CONCLUSION

Professionalism is now an integral part of medical curricula and assessment processes, and the subject is considered in selection processes at both basic (undergraduate and postgraduate) and specialty levels of entry. This is not an easy task, especially in that definitions and the understanding of professionalism is itself changing. Improvements in communication, increased public awareness and other societal changes have resulted in greater public understanding of both the importance of professionalism and what constitutes poor professionalism. Although 'sound' professionalism is much the same in an increasingly globalised 'health industry', complexities arise when national borders are crossed, largely because of differences in culture, religion, health and legal systems. Dealing with cases of poor professionalism remains a challenge everywhere; hence, this book.

REFERENCES

1. West MA. *Effective Teamwork: practical lessons from organizational research.* 3rd ed. Chichester: Wiley-Blackwell; 2012.
2. Wilson R McL, Runciman WB, Gibberd RW, *et al.* The Quality in Australian Health Care Study. *Med J Aust.* 1995; **163**(9): 458–71.
3. McGlynn EA, Steven M, Asch SM, *et al.* The quality of health care delivered to adults in the United States. *N Engl J Med.* 2003; **348**(26):2635–45.
4. Rowe N. Health and safety legislation and the NHS. *Clin Risk.* 2006; **12**(5): 207–8.
5. Borges NJ, Manuel RS, Elam CL, *et al.* Differences in motives between Millennial and Generation X medical students. *Med Educ.* 2010; **44**(6): 570–6.
6. Legal Careers. *Generation X.* Available at: http://legalcareers.about.com/od/practicetips/a/GenerationX.htm (accessed 8 May 2013).
7. English Online. *Generation Y: their attitudes towards work and life.* Available at: www.english-online.at/news-articles/living/generation-y-their-attitudes-toward-life-and-work.htm (accessed 8 May 2013).
8. Kind T, Genrich G, Doshi A, *et al.* Social media policies at US medical schools. *Med Educ Online.* 2010; **15**: 5324–31. Available at: http://med-ed-online.net/index.php/meo/article/view/5324 (accessed 15 February 2013).
9. Australian Medical Association Council of Doctors-in-training; New Zealand Medical Association Doctors-in-training Council, New Zealand Medical Students'

Association; Australian Medical Students' Association. *Social Media and the Medical Profession: a guide to online professionalism for medical practitioners and medical students.* November 2010. Available at: https://ama.com.au/social-media-and-medical-profession (accessed 8 May 2013).

10. Merzel C, D'Afflitti J. Reconsidering community-based health promotion: promise, performance, and potential. *Am J Public Health.* 2003; **93**(4): 557–74.

11. Bandi P, Cokkinides V, Smith RA, *et al.* Trends in colorectal cancer screening with home-based fecal occult blood tests in adults aged 50 to 64 years, 2000–2008. *Cancer.* 2013; **118**(20): 5092–9.

12. Health Workforce New Zealand. *Training intentions.* Available at: www.healthwork force.govt.nz/tools-and-resources/for-employers-educators/hwnz-training-intentions (accessed 8 May 2013).

13. Bristol Royal Infirmary Inquiry. *The Inquiry into the Management of Care of Children Undergoing Complex Heart Surgery at the Bristol Royal Infirmary.* Command Paper CM 5207. London: HMSO; 2001. Available at: http://webarchive.nationalarchives.gov. uk/20090811143745/http://www.bristol-inquiry.org.uk (accessed 8 May 2013).

14. Queensland Health. *Bundaberg Hospital Commission of Enquiry.* Queensland: Queensland Government; 2005. Available at: www.health.qld.gov.au/inquiry/docs/inquiry.pdf (accessed 15 February 2013).

15. Department of Health. *The Shipman Inquiry.* London: Her Majesty's Stationery Office; 2005. Available at: http://webarchive.nationalarchives.gov.uk/20060715141954/http://the-shipman-inquiry.org.uk/home.asp (accessed 8 May 2013).

16. Mid Staffordshire NHS Foundation Trust Inquiry. *Robert Francis Inquiry Report into Mid-Staffordshire NHS Foundation Trust.* London: Department of Health; 2013. Available at: http://webarchive.nationalarchives.gov.uk/20130107105354/http://www.dh.gov. uk/en/Publicationsandstatistics/Publications/PublicationsPolicyAndGuidance/DH_113018 (accessed 8 May 2013).

17. World Federation of Medical Education. Quality improvement in basic medical education. Copenhagen: WFME; 2012. Available at: www.wfme.org/standards/bme (accessed 8 May 2013).

18. Papadakis M, Hodgson CS, Teherani A, *et al.* Unprofessional behavior in medical school is associated with subsequent disciplinary action by a state medical board. *Acad Med.* 2004; **79**(3): 244–9.

19. Eva KW, Rosenfeld J, Reiter HI, *et al.* An admissions OSCE: the multiple mini-interview. *Med Educ.* 2004; **38**(3): 314–26.

CHAPTER 5

Public policy and the patient: professionalism and regulation – a UK perspective

Professionalism is important in terms of promoting good standards of practice, but the public policy aspects of professionalism also need to be discussed, including the role played by regulators. The focus in this chapter is on the patient rather than the doctor.

Regulation is everyone's business, and it is not just the concern of the professionals who are being regulated, or of policy experts and governments. It is, or should be, part of a wider endeavour, and to be effective it should engage with the public and reflect societal trends and ways of thinking. The mechanics of the process may be the reserve of specialist advisors and members of governing councils and committees, but those charged with responsibility for effective regulation do need to engage with the wider public in order to fulfil the remit of providing a proper public service.

Members of any profession, whether medicine, law, teaching, social work or anything else, are there to serve the public, and the moment members of those professions lose that focus and look after their own interests instead, problems tend to occur. It is partly a question of how those charged with the responsibility of regulating a profession such as medicine go about the task, and partly a question of establishing a dialogue and engaging with the public (which ought not to be difficult in an era of rapid communication). In the twenty-first century there is no need for regulation and public policy to be iconoclastic – many (although not all) of its functions can be open and accountable, and in this chapter we consider professionalism from the points of view of public policy, medical regulation and the patient.

This chapter has a focus on the United Kingdom, partly for reasons to do with familiarity and first-hand experience, and partly because without anchoring discussion to a particular place and healthcare system it would simply be too easy to lapse into generalities. This would be tedious and unedifying, and besides which, policy comparison across international boundaries is a challenging and technical task. Even within the four countries that make up the United Kingdom there are difficulties in making systems work nationally while still being sensitive to local needs and differences in law, so to compare public policy on health regulation between Australia, New Zealand, the United States and the United Kingdom would require more time, space and effort than would be appropriate for a book such as this. While there are certainly common elements between these countries in terms of language and culture, there are significant differences in law, politics, economics and public administration, each of which potentially affects how regulation works in practice.

For instance, colleagues in New Zealand describe the most important procedural issues as being the regular longitudinal monitoring of student progress through meetings of relevant staff at several stages during each year, and a system of 'conditional pass' that results in staff finding it easier to raise issues even if they are unsure of the validity of such concerns. Any student for whom there are concerns about performance or who obtains a conditional pass meets the associate dean for student affairs so that more information can be gathered and considered. As a consequence, the system is more sensitive than specific in identifying concerns. In other words, a number of the problems picked up by this system turn out to be 'false positives' where, following investigation or further follow-up, no major problems actually emerged. Colleagues in New Zealand regard this as preferable to a system that produces too many 'false negatives', whereby students who have problems with professional behaviours might otherwise be missed. Their second tier of referral is the Fitness to Practise Committee, and if problems are found to be serious and/or irremediable, then the committee considers the circumstances and can recommend failure or exclusion from the course, further intervention or, in the case of health concerns, notification to the Medical Council of New Zealand.[1-3],*

PROFESSIONAL REGULATION

In the last decade the United Kingdom has seen a number of changes in medical professional regulation, and this process of change is continuing. This is healthy and necessary even if it creates a potential problem for commentators and analysts, because by the time a book such as this is in print, things could

---

* Our thanks to T Wilkinson and J McKenzie for providing this information.

have already changed. That said, the fundamental issues tend to remain the same, and one of the main challenges facing regulators is about being able to protect the public, helping them to have confidence in their doctors while at the same time making sure that systems employed in carrying out necessary tasks are fair and not overly burdensome.

The risks of failure are twofold: if the public loses confidence in the system then government may be forced to step in, and if doctors themselves lose confidence in the regulator then the system could become unworkable. While it is unsurprising if doctors sometimes feel that the regulator is hostile towards them, or if they perceive the regulator to be unable to understand their needs and concerns, doctors should not get sanctioned without the case first having been through an extensive process of assessment and independent review. No system is foolproof, but trivial or malicious cases ought not to progress that far. More to the point, if a regulator lacks the power to operate effectively, or if it lacks the resources to do a proper job in protecting the public from a doctor whose clinical performance or professional behaviour fails to meet the standards expected, it will lack public respect and will therefore be failing in its primary mission.

Doctors are sometimes known to express frustration at having to pay an annual fee in order to stay on the medical register, but the General Medical Council (GMC) is neither a club nor a trades union, like the British Medical Association, which doctors can choose to belong to or not. Medical regulation is binding, and therefore no registration means not having the right to practise medicine (or at least not in the United Kingdom). It is the price of self-regulation to sign up (and pay up) to a social contract arrangement that allows the profession to regulate itself without undue interference from central government. That a government will communicate with a regulator is fair and reasonable, but with a social contract arrangement, central government should not dictate policy or impose its will, unless it first wants to bring about a change in the law.[4]

A lively debate is going on in the United Kingdom at the time of writing to do with self-regulation, ethics and the press. The outcome of an extensive (and expensive) public inquiry was published in late 2012,[5] and this involved a detailed report on past major lapses in (if not a total disregard for) standards and ethics by sections of the press. A similar process occurred with doctors in 2004–05 when Dame Janet Smith published her report into affairs relating to the late Dr Harold Shipman, following a public inquiry into failures in administration and systems of medical regulation. Systems that were in force had proved inadequate for the task and unable to prevent a family physician from killing many patients and going undetected for an extensive period of time.[6]

While the outcome of that debate stopped short of a new statute, it led to,

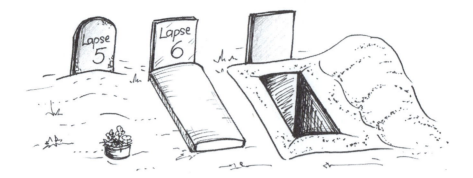

among other things, significant reorganisations within the GMC. This included the introduction of a 50:50 split in the composition of the Council between lay and medical, so that while doctors were allowed to continue to regulate themselves, they now do so with active participation from representative members of the public. Whether perceived or actual, 'doctors looking after doctors' or 'lawyers looking after lawyers' is no longer seen as publicly acceptable without additional measures to satisfy public demands for a voice of its own and greater accountability. 'Light-touch regulation' is a phrase that was once popular with politicians, but it has a downside, and when applied to banking it triggered consequences in the world of finance that still resonate around the world.

An intelligent approach to regulation has to be balanced. In short, too much regulation inhibits freedoms and is expensive to administer; too little regulation and the public lacks protection, whether from doctors, lawyers, journalists, bankers or any other group of professionals that fails to meet public expectations in terms of standards and ethics. Later in this chapter we consider practical aspects of how the UK medical regulator tackles the issue of professionalism, but first we need to consider professionalism and public policy from the point of view of the medical educator.

PROFESSIONALISM AND MEDICAL EDUCATION

How doctors behave as practising professionals *could* be influenced by how they behaved as medical students; attitudes and behaviours that prevail in later life could start in the early stages of someone's career, although that is not necessarily the case. In Chapter 2 we referred to the work of Papadakis and others[7] who explore links between the behaviour of medical students and the behaviour of qualified doctors; the task here is not to look for causal connections or 'proof', but rather to examine professionalism in medical education from the point of view of public policy.

Medical students are doctors in training, and while they are not yet providing a service to patients on their own, they certainly have a degree of responsibility for providing patient care. While a medical student's personal responsibility may be limited, with accountability resting mainly with the clinician in charge, student behaviours certainly affect others, including patients and peers. As in the case studies in Part Two, we see that a small number of medical students do behave in inappropriate and regrettable ways; while this is often damaging to careers, it has much wider implications in terms of medical education and policies that are designed to protect the general public.

In Chapter 2 we explained our reasoning as to why we think it is important for doctors to be taught and assessed in professionalism during the full course of their training; here we consider why we believe that *policy* implications arise in the context of teaching, training and assessing professionalism. The reasons are threefold:

1. Medical education concerns the public at large; it is more than just something that doctors go through in order to qualify and become registered – it defines who doctors are as people, including how they work and how they interact with patients and other professionals. Unprofessional students and trainees can turn into unprofessional qualified doctors if problem behaviours are not spotted and/or remediated. Effective sanctions need to be in place to stop someone progressing to the point of graduation, or completing his or her medical training in cases where significant problems with professional behaviours persist.

2. Medical degrees are portable, and doctors can easily train in one country and go work in another; given considerable differences in terms of if, when and how doctors acquire skills in professionalism, as well as wide differences in the culture of healthcare itself, doctors' attitudes can have a direct impact on the standard of care provided in the community where they work. Given that attitudes typically precede behaviours, professionalism is something that medical schools and postgraduate colleges need to take seriously. (However, this is not always the case, and in countries such as India, which trains a large number of doctors, professionalism is rarely either taught or assessed.)[8]

3. The idea of medical practice as a form of public service is something that tends to fade during the course of someone's medical career, either on account of early role model influences or perhaps because of growing awareness that what happens in everyday clinical practice fails to live up to expectations and former ideals about altruism and public service; growing personal maturity and insights arising from personal experience may or may not be sufficient to be able to counter these influences.

Professionalism demands an element of accountability being shown by educators towards members of the public, which relies on having access to a trained, skilled workforce. The public has an interest in workforce training simply to help ensure the provision of healthcare services into the future, even if this has to be tempered by what society can afford and how much of that cost should be borne by a student or trainee. Once doctors are registered and qualified, it is largely their responsibility to pay for advanced medical education, but initial training attracts an element of subsidy, especially in a healthcare system such as the British National Health Service that is funded primarily out of central taxation.

If medicine as a profession is seen as being too self-serving, it calls into question whether any public subsidy should be involved in medical education, especially having in mind potential future earnings from being a doctor. For these reasons, the policy aspects of medical education should not be ignored (even if programmes are run by or in collaboration with privately run institutions).[9–12] The patient (as a member of the public) is a key stakeholder in the enterprise of training the workforce and the provision of quality, safe medical care.

PUBLIC POLICY

Issues around public protection and patient safety have a relatively high profile in each of the countries covered by this book, and governments often have dedicated agencies for monitoring patient safety and quality of care, such as the Health Quality and Safety Commission in New Zealand, or the Health Protection Agency or Care Quality Commission in the United Kingdom.[13–15] Weak regulation, for instance, can lead to poor monitoring of infection rates and poor standards of safety in hospitals, which potentially puts the public at risk, which is another reason why regulation in healthcare should be seen as being everyone's business. The ease and accessibility of data on infection control in the United Kingdom, for instance, is a practical example of a public policy aimed at helping communities to rely on having safe, quality care.[16]

Failures in professionalism may not have the same profile as failures to provide good clinical care, but in our view, it is a mistake to think that the two are not linked. Poor standards of professionalism easily result in poor standards of care; for instance, a trainee doctor who consistently turns up late for work could be putting patients at risk because of inadequate levels of staffing (unless another doctor is willing and able to provide cover). Furthermore, doctors who do not respect proper boundaries in terms of sexual relationships put patients and colleagues at risk by reason of their inappropriate behaviours, and doctors who abuse drugs are unlikely to be able to perform at their best. Such problems are rare but not rare enough, and without powerful sanctions arising from effective regulation, public protection mechanisms may not be up to the task of ensuring adequate patient safety.

In terms of setting public policy, there is a variety of methods for promoting patient and public involvement in healthcare policy setting, which includes:

- the use of public consultations
- open meetings, workshops and other fora involving non-medics and interested members of the public
- lay representation on committees and councils (e.g. having an even split between lay and professional membership)
- active engagement with the 'third' sector, with representatives from charities being invited to comment on draft policies
- active engagement with people directly affected by new policies but who are potentially disenfranchised because of socio-economic factors that hinder their participation (known as hard-to-reach groups).

A range of consultation methods, including patient and public involvement, for instance, was employed in 2007–10 when the GMC was developing regulatory policy on professional behaviours and medical students' fitness to practise medicine (the guidance that ensued from it being particularly relevant to this discussion).[17] All this is worthwhile even if it is expensive and time-consuming, and in an organisation such as the GMC, it is now a routine part of the process of developing standards and setting regulation policy.[18]

This level of lay participation and public consultation is perhaps less often employed in the context of setting education policy, since education policy decisions are normally taken locally by universities, heads of medical schools and/or National Health Service managers, or nationally by the Medical Schools Council or in conjunction with the Department of Health.[19] While not all aspects of medical education policy involve public participation, the public clearly has an interest in the outcome of the process, to say nothing about its investment through the provision of public subsidy, which is something that policymakers need to keep in mind.

WORKFORCE PLANNING

Once a student graduates, he or she becomes part of the workforce, and some ethical issues arise around workforce planning and professionalism. Governments and healthcare providers have to consider supply and demand in the workforce. First, if too *few* doctors are trained it leads to workforce shortages; second, when doctors have been trained it can be hard getting them to work in poorer neighbourhoods and/or remote rural locations. Conversely, if too *many* doctors are trained it creates problems for new graduates trying to find training places, and it is also wasteful in terms of the use of public resources. In that it takes 10 years to train new doctors, population health needs always need to be met, and so the public ought at least to have a say.

Ensuring an adequate supply of doctors in poorer neighbourhoods and remote rural locations is challenging, and as a policy issue it comes up against freedom of choice and the individual autonomy of the doctor. Although the United Kingdom does not have bush country or indigenous populations with complex health needs living in outback regions hundreds of miles from a town, it has a problem to the extent that not all doctors want to work in inner cities, or go work in the Welsh hills or the Scottish Highlands. An ethical issue exists with regard to how much weight to give to doctor autonomy (i.e. in terms of career) compared with meeting public and population needs. Allowing qualified doctors to work in areas where *they* want to live potentially leads to gaps in service provision, just as allowing doctors the freedom to choose their specialty (i.e. immediately after the period of initial training) can lead to gaps in relation to the provision of general practice. While some developing countries adopt coercive methods to help address these problems, this does not apply to the United Kingdom, even though the professionalism of junior doctors could well be challenged if they are *required* to go and work in unpopular areas.

Nonetheless, the system overall works reasonably well, and while not all doctors may like the eventual outcome, it offers a workable and balanced arrangement in terms of public policy and meeting the needs of the population. However, one could go further and pursue the notion that it would be 'unprofessional' for a graduate to leave an area of workforce need and move to the city (with better schools, higher income and potential for private practice), and 'unprofessional' to decline a specialty training post in an undersubscribed specialty in favour of somewhere more 'glamorous'. This might be a step too far, and enforcing such an approach would be legally challenging and restrictive of professional autonomy, even though it forms part of the debate about professional responsibility and service to the community. To coerce clinicians to work in areas of greatest need unavoidably means pitching population needs directly against the career aspirations of trainee doctors; an alternative approach would be to encourage doctors to be mindful of the *moral* value of providing care in underserved (geographic or clinical) areas as a way of balancing public and private interest, perhaps for a limited period of time; we know that some doctors do take this seriously and allow this thought to influence their choices, but this is not always the case.

Just prior to graduation, UK doctors apply to a number of education centres (currently known as deaneries), and while they are allowed to state an order of preference, the process of matching applicants to places is ultimately performed by means of computer allocation. The choice of specialty comes *after* completing basic training, which normally lasts for 2 years, and it is at that stage that supply and demand become much more of an issue. If too many doctors want to become surgeons, for instance, they might not succeed in finding training places, and therefore have to consider choosing other less popular specialties, such as obstetrics and gynaecology, or anaesthetics.

To continue with this staged approach, the aspiring doctor has gained a medical degree, been through basic training and embarked on a programme of specialty training (in conjunction with one of the medical colleges), whether or not his or her personal motivation is altruistic; it is at this point, perhaps, that the focus of attention needs to shift towards maintaining standards of professionalism throughout the later stages of a doctor's career.*

PROFESSIONALISM AND REVALIDATION

Because of its public role, a regulatory body such as the GMC is well aware of the importance of professionalism, and it has already been noted how the organisation went to some lengths in drawing up guidance for medical students, but the same issues are just as important for the fully qualified, registered, doctor. Because of this importance attaching to professionalism, various policy initiatives have resulted in an extensive period of debate on how best to try to ensure *prospectively* that doctors adhere to the standards of professionalism that are expected of them.[20,21] This process eventually resulted in the introduction of a system of revalidation in 2012, and that now applies to all doctors carrying full registration. Nobody knows whether or not a system whereby doctors have to provide evidence of their standards of competence will prove to be effective in protecting the public and rooting out 'dangerous doctors', but a build-up of public pressure effectively meant that a formal system of quality assurance had to be put in place in order to try to boost public confidence in the profession.

To quote from the GMC:

> Revalidation is the process by which licensed doctors are required to demonstrate on a regular basis that they are up to date and fit to practise. Revalidation aims to give extra confidence to patients that their doctor is being regularly checked by their employer and the GMC.[22]

Nobody can be sure that regulatory insights into professionalism will be sufficient to satisfy demands for action (from government and the public) in providing meaningful information about a doctor's professional standards,

---

* For further comments on workforce planning *see* Chapter 4.

and no data on the effectiveness of revalidation is likely to be available before at least 2014. However, that such a system has been put in place is itself evidence that professionalism and public accountability go hand in hand and that self-regulation encompasses quality control measures that go beyond issues of basic clinical competence.

For example, medical students graduating from UK schools now have to pass a situational judgement test that assesses their ability to think clearly and rationally and to correctly identify professional issues; this has little to do with technical knowledge or expertise, but it has much to do with how a doctor thinks and how that doctor might conduct him- or herself in the future in different clinical situations.[23]

UNPROFESSIONAL BEHAVIOURS AND FITNESS TO PRACTISE (OR PROGRESS)*

At one stage we considered an alternative title for this book: *'Doctors behaving badly and what to do about it'*. It is clear that doctors do occasionally step out of line and display a range of unprofessional and even criminal behaviours. There are sufficient cases of professional misconduct presented in Part Two to illustrate the point that doctors and trainees sometimes behave badly and need to be sanctioned, but this is the exception rather than the general rule. Most doctors behave professionally most of the time; but those who do not sometimes fail miserably.

While student problems are generally dealt with 'in-house', matters do not stop there, and when students graduate in the United Kingdom they have to make a self-declaration about their 'fitness to practise', stating whether or not they have had an encounter with conduct committees or disciplinary panels of inquiry. Additionally, when a qualified doctor is investigated by the GMC for allegations of misconduct, it is not uncommon for the regulator to contact the medical school where a doctor trained in order to find out relevant information that might be contained in the student record. This means that information is sometimes shared, and student misdemeanours do not necessarily stay in the student domain.

Postgraduate misdemeanours are not judged against different criteria; there

---

* A medical student or trainee is assessed according to whether or not he or she is considered fit to move on and progress to the next level. While the terminology differs as well as the systems used to assess professional competence, the outcomes are broadly similar in so far as a student or trainee who fails to satisfy the relevant criteria and who is found unsuited to be able to progress to the higher level will be held back, subject to appropriate sanctions or required to leave the programme. Both systems are meant to address public safety and protection, although they go about the task slightly differently. Differences also apply in respect of systems used for assessing professional competence in Australia and New Zealand.

is an element of linkage between student, trainee and fully qualified doctor performance, especially where serious problems arise, even though the expectations from a first-year medical student will differ somewhat from those of a doctor with 5 or 10 years' clinical experience. The criteria for students and qualified professionals, as set out in core GMC guidance called *Good Medical Practice*,[24] are applicable in equal measure to both groups.

Regulatory systems that operate in the United Kingdom mean that for doctors in training, unprofessional conduct will usually be dealt with first at local level (i.e. by their employers). Even cases referred directly to the GMC can be referred back to local service providers to be dealt with if there is no major element of public interest. On the other hand, adjudications that are sufficiently serious as to involve the regulator need to take place more within the public domain. Such cases are eventually heard before members of the Medical Practitioners Tribunal Service (MPTS), and while this body falls under the general auspices of the GMC, it is independently run.[25] The outcome of recent cases heard by the MPTS are 'open access', and so anybody can go online to see a transcript or look up the status of a doctor on the GMC register and see if there are any conditions attached to his or her medical registration.[26]

There is inevitably an element of public scrutiny when cases are heard before a tribunal, and privacy and confidentially cannot be maintained when the point is reached that a case warrants a full hearing. Furthermore, if a finding goes against a doctor who is being investigated, the full transcript then becomes a matter of public record. There are some checks and balances, however, that exist *after* a case has been decided; for instance a doctor can try to overturn an MPTS decision by appealing to the High Court, and cases can be subject to additional layers of scrutiny via a body known as the Professional Standards Authority.[27] Whether these systems work effectively and fulfil the task of providing adequate protection to the public while being fair to the individual clinician is open for debate, because the current arrangements are still relatively new. However, there is no adequate reason for doubting their effectiveness, and the system has a layer of independent scrutiny.

Overall, while the structures outlined in this chapter are complex and subject to regular review and periods of reform, this commentary illustrates how public policy works in one of the countries that we write about in this book. It should therefore provide a suitable backdrop to help readers make sense of the cases that follow in Part Two.

REFERENCES

1. Wilkinson TJ, Tweed M, Egan T, *et al.* Joining the dots: conditional pass and programmatic assessment enhances recognition of problems with professionalism and factors hampering student progress. *BMC Med Educ.* 2011; **11**: 29.

2. University of Otago Faculty of Medicine. *Code of Practice for Fitness to Practise.* Dunedin: University of Otago; 2010. Available at: http://micn.otago.ac.nz/wp-content/uploads/micn/2008/03/Code-of-Practice-for-Fitness-to-Practice-2010.pdf (accessed 17 February 2013).

3. University of Otago. *Dishonest Practice Procedures.* Dunedin: University of Otago; 2011. Available at: www.otago.ac.nz/administration/policies/otago003145.html (accessed 17 February 2013).

4. Medical Act 1983. Available at: www.legislation.gov.uk/ukpga/1983/54/section/35C (accessed 9 May 2013).

5. The Leveson Report. *An Inquiry into the Culture, Practices and Ethics of the Press: report [Leveson].* London: TSO; 2012. Available at: www.official-documents.gov.uk/document/ hc1213/hc07/0780/0780.asp (accessed 2 February 2013).

6. Department of Health. *The Shipman Inquiry.* London: Her Majesty's Stationery Office; 2005. Available at: http://webarchive.nationalarchives.gov.uk/20060715141954/ http://the-shipman-inquiry.org.uk/home.asp (accessed 9 May 2013).

7. Papadakis MA, Hodgson CS, Tehrani A, *et al.* Unprofessional behavior in medical school is associated with subsequent disciplinary action by a state medical board. *Acad Med.* 2004; **79**(3): 244–9.

8. Worthington RP. Medicine, ethics and professionalism in modern India. In: Worthington RP, Rohrbaugh RM. *Health Policy and Ethics: a critical examination of values from a global perspective.* London: Radcliffe Publishing; 2011. pp. 72–5.

9. Dorsey ER, Nicholson S, Frist W. Commentary: improving the supply and distribution of primary care physicians. *Acad Med.* 2011; **86**(5): 541–3.

10. Newhouse JP, Wilensky GR. Paying for graduate medical education: the debate goes on. *Health Aff (Millwood).* 2001; **20**(2): 136–47.

11. Rosenthal J, Stephenson A. General practice: the future teaching environment: a report on undergraduate primary care education in London. *Br J Gen Pract.* 2010; **60**(571): 144.

12. Murray E, Jinks V, Modell M. Community-based medical education: feasibility and cost. *Med Educ.* 1995; **29**(1): 66–71.

13. New Zealand Health Quality and Safety Commission. *About the Commission.* Available at: www.hqsc.govt.nz/about-the-commission/ (accessed 9 May 2013).

14. www.hpa.org.uk/HPAwebHome/

15. www.cqc.org.uk/

16. Public Health England. *Mandatory Surveillance Weekly Reports.* Available at: www. hpa.org.uk/Topics/InfectiousDiseases/InfectionsAZ/StaphylococcusAureus/ EpidemiologicalData/MandatorySurveillance/hcaimrsaandcdiweeklyreports/ (accessed 9 May 2013).

17. General Medical Council. *Medical Students: professional values and fitness to practise.* London: GMC; 2010. Available at: www.gmc-uk.org/education/undergraduate/ professional_behaviour.asp (accessed 2 February 2013).

18. General Medical Council (UK). *Consultations.* Available at: www.gmc-uk.org/about/ consultations.asp (accessed 9 May 2013).

19. UK Medical Schools Council. *Information.* Available at: www.medschools.ac.uk/ AboutUs/Pages/default.aspx (accessed 9 May 2013).

20. Southgate L, Pringle M. Revalidation in the United Kingdom: general principles based

on experience in general practice. *Br Med J*. 1999; **319**(7218): 1180–3. Available at: www.ncbi.nlm.nih.gov/pmc/articles/PMC1116961/ (accessed 2 February 2013).

21. Irvine D. Patients, professionalism, and revalidation. *Br Med J*. 2005; **330**(7502): 1265–8. Available at: www.ncbi.nlm.nih.gov/pmc/articles/PMC558103/ (accessed 2 February 2013).

22. General Medical Council (UK). *Revalidation*. Available at: www.gmc-uk.org/doctors/revalidation.asp (accessed 9 May 2013).

23. NHS Foundation Programme. *Home*. Available at: www.foundationprogramme.nhs.uk/pages/home/how-to-apply (accessed 9 May 2013).

24. General Medical Council. *Good Medical Practice (2013)*. London: GMC; 2006. Available at: www.gmc-uk.org/guidance/good_medical_practice.asp (accessed 2 February 2013).

25. Medical Practitioners Tribunal Service. *Decisions*. Available at: www.mpts-uk.org/decisions/1421.asp (accessed 9 May 2013).

26. General Medical Council (UK). *List of Registered Medical Practitioners*. Available at: www.gmc-uk.org/doctors/register/LRMP.asp (accessed 9 May 2013).

27. Professional Standards Authority. *Our Work*. Available at: www.professionalstandards.org.uk/about-us/our-work (accessed 9 May 2013).

Part Two

Case studies

INTRODUCTION

Part Two presents a series of cases gathered from the United States, the United Kingdom, New Zealand and Australia that demonstrate the real, 'messy' world of how cases of poor professionalism present and are managed. All cases are based on real episodes, and in some cases a combination of real episodes, but they have been appropriately de-identified. Local jurisdictional and contextual information is provided because it influences precisely how cases must be managed; there are many similarities, but also some key differences, in how health professional regulation of students and recent graduates is applied even in nations with apparently similar health systems and legal frameworks. Furthermore, a medical school in one jurisdiction may have different systems and regulations from a medical school in another jurisdiction, with different nomenclature for processes and structures. Where applicable we, as editors, have kept 'local' nomenclature.

Some elements of the cases may seem hard to believe and too far-fetched; however, if anything, the more complex cases have been simplified for ease of reading rather than the opposite, and complexity was never added in just for effect. Readers may note that some types of unprofessional behaviour occur much more frequently than others, but that is based on direct experience. Cases not infrequently involve drug abuse or addiction; also, there is clearly a gender bias in relation to the subjects of each case, and in both instances this is borne out by fact, i.e. in terms of cases coming before committees and presenting themselves to the contributor authors.

More cases of unprofessional conduct tend to arise involving young men than young women, and we would be distorting the facts unnecessarily if we were to change genders out of respect for notions of equality. Equality of process is what matters, and that men and women are both treated fairly; if more male doctors and medical students come before disciplinary committees and panels than female, that may simply be how it is. We should also add that if any cases closely resemble cases that are known to a reader, that is purely unintentional, unless, however, we refer to a case that is in the public domain, and in which case we try to make that clear. Where that does arise, then we have fictionalised so as not to mirror actual cases too closely. Every case has elements of truth, and while some are more imaginatively constructed than others, none are pure fiction.

All the cases are designed to provoke discussion among groups of learners, and it is likely that readers may think of additional questions and pursue additional discussion points as they adapt cases to their own specific contexts. The cases are organised into chapters along geographical lines, and within the chapters they are grouped according to content. Individual headings provide a flavour of what the case is about, and the format for each case is standard. Each case begins with an outline description that provides the narrative part of the case, followed by a list of questions to be considered, a discussion section and a summary of key points. This summary is formulated as a set of responses to a standardised list of questions.

1. Which elements do you see as being most important in terms of professionalism, and were the issues properly addressed?
2. Was the outcome fair and just (in your view); if not, in what way and on whom do you think it was unfair?
3. To what extent is the case about patient safety and public protection?
4. What lessons can be learned from the case in terms of education and training?
5. Was protocol an issue and what lessons can the institution learn?
6. Are there any issues that should concern the regulator and not just local educators?
7. Were local and/or national guidelines utilised and, if so, were they fit for purpose?

CHAPTER 6

The United Kingdom and the United States

CASE STUDIES 1–15
CASE 1

A first-year postgraduate doctor known for having 'Monday morning-itis'.

Outline

SE, A 25-year-old Foundation year 1 doctor, appears to have a pattern of late attendance, especially on Monday mornings. She is often 1–2 hours late and seems tired and inattentive, with low work efficiency until after lunch. Her colleagues make jokes such as 'you must have had quite a weekend!' Repeated instances over two different terms causes concern for her consultants, and one consultant tries to discuss the matter with her, but SE avoids the topic, simply saying that she is 'not a Monday person' and that it takes her a while to settle into work. She denies that there are any other problems; however, there are rumours that she is often seen at all-night parties on weekends and that she is a frequent user of Ecstasy and cannabis. She is referred to the programme director in order to discuss her progress.

At this meeting the programme director directly raises concerns about drug use and safety at work. Under pressure, SE admits that she often uses cannabis and Ecstasy, but only on weekends in her 'own time', and that she will sometimes drink alcohol as well, but that there is always a 'clear 8 hours' between drug consumption and starting work – 'like airline pilots'. She therefore feels that she is in full control and is not addicted to any drugs – she just enjoys them as they enhance the party experience. She says that this is no different from her colleagues drinking alcohol – generally much more than she does

– at social events, citing research that appears to suggest that intermittent use of these drugs causes no long-term health effects. She does not believe that she poses any risk to patient safety on Monday mornings, or indeed at any other time. The programme director is concerned on two grounds: the first is that SE is involved in risk-taking behaviour and the second is that she appears to have impaired insight.

The risks are probably greater than she states, and there is evidence from peers and colleagues that her performance is affected, largely on account of a disturbed sleep pattern after using drugs. Particularly worrying is her reluctance to change the behaviour, and the programme director has no choice but to refer her to the General Medical Council (GMC). As part of the preliminary investigation she is required to undertake a full health assessment by an independent medical examiner, the findings of which indicate that there is indeed a problem. Her case is not referred to the Medical Practitioners Tribunal Service,[1] but she is given notice that she must work under supervision and be tested for illegal drug use at regular intervals, giving an undertaking that she will cease using cannabis and Ecstasy.

After 3 months, random drug screening tests show traces of cannabis on two separate occasions. SE is told either to accept having her licence to practise suspended and face a full investigation by the Medical Practitioners Tribunal Service or to agree to enrolling immediately on a drug rehabilitation programme and then to continue with supervised registration for a period of 6 months. If she is not 'clean' after this time, she will lose her place on the Foundation Programme and she will be automatically assessed for fitness to practise, which could potentially mean permanent erasure from the medical register.

Questions

- Is it right that use of cannabis, Ecstasy and other recreational drugs are treated differently from alcohol use?
- What is the role of regulators in managing behaviours outside the workplace, and when should behaviours trigger a process of regulatory review?
- In essence, is this a health problem, a professionalism issue, or both?
- How easily can drug use be monitored, and what is the likely prognosis in a case such as this?

Discussion

The use of class A and B drugs[2] by professionals is an interesting issue in that legal implications for ordinary citizens are relatively minor. The expectation of health professionals is not the same as for the general public, and the extent to which this difference is justifiable is worth considering. When the GMC updates its guidance it engages in a wide process of patient and public engagement. While opinions will vary, a consensus position has to be reached about the rights of doctors to a private life, and explanatory notes supporting the 2013 edition of *Good Medical Practice* state that 'doctors must make sure that their conduct at all times justifies their patients' trust in them and the public's trust in the profession'.[3] While doctors are neither more nor less than a (specially trained) section of the general public, expectations in terms of their behaviour may well be different. This is not just a question of public attitude; it is also about patient safety and public protection, and if a doctor is engaging in the type of behaviour shown by SE, the public has reason to be concerned and so the regulator needs to be involved. Soon SE will have greater levels of responsibility, and it is simply not acceptable that her ability to function is impaired in this way, especially because it occurs on a regular basis; for her own sake as well as that of her patients, she needs expert help.

Her supervisor acted appropriately in referring her for preliminary investigations; her lack of insight into her unprofessional conduct is troublesome, the criminal nature of her behaviour notwithstanding. As we note in Chapter 8, drug use by doctors may not be as unusual as one would wish, and regulators around the world have had to find effective ways to try to deal with this issue.

SE's point about alcohol use is not without foundation. Both forms of abuse are harmful, although perhaps in different ways. We do not have the expertise to comment on the science of addiction, although we recognise that abuse of alcohol can be detrimental to the health of doctors and patients alike.

Whether the associated harms of drug as opposed to alcohol abuse are equally worthy of public condemnation is a matter for debate, and in that ethical standards primarily reflect what society is prepared to tolerate at a given point in time, subject to limits imposed by law, then the issue may be more about law than morality or professional standards. From time to time Parliament considers these issues, and the classification (or declassification) of drugs is a matter for politicians and their advisors.[4]

Questions of monitoring are important in this case, and without monitoring the regulator can do no more than take doctors at their word, which, as we know, is not always sufficient. Doctors (and others) sometimes go to great lengths in order to try to disguise 'problem behaviours', including lying to a regulator, and so an objective means of testing has to be part of the process of remediation and rehabilitation. Furthermore, urine screening for cannabis is rather imprecise about the timing of the use, showing positive results up to 13 days after the last cannabis use. Given that SE did not manage to break her habit, and lapses showed that she continued using at least one illegal drug, then it is entirely appropriate that she is presented with the stark choice: 'go on to rehabilitation now or be suspended and face a full investigation'.

Summary

- Lack of insight into the nature of the problem was an important part of this case, as well as her unwillingness to change her behaviour.
- Clinical educators and regulators have to balance the need for justice with wider responsibilities to the public; without strong measures, the situation with SE could otherwise have gone unchecked.
- Patient safety and public protection are central to this case, trumping individual freedoms.
- Educators need to know when to be supportive and when to escalate a case; suitable training should help with developing these skills.
- Protocol was followed, and having robust procedures should help to ensure that events follow the right course.
- The regulator will generally have more experience in dealing with these issues than local educators; their involvement in this case was crucial.
- GMC guidelines provide a valuable framework and help ensure fairness to the individual, while simultaneously protecting the public from doctors who may be unsafe.

CASE 2

A medical student is caught selling 'balloons' on campus.

Outline

A security officer notices TW, a final-year medical student, to be inflating balloons with nitrous oxide and inhaling the gas at a university concert. This attracts the attention of other students, a few of whom buy canisters and balloons from TW and inhale the gas themselves. He is expelled from the venue and a report of the incident finds its way from the security office to the registrar's office, and then to the head of the school of medicine. The report is critical of the student, using terms such as 'drug trafficking', 'poor role modelling' and 'bringing the university into disrepute'. The whole school soon hears all about the incident, and TW is called in for an interview with the head of school. During the interview TW apologises profusely, but he expresses surprise that the behaviour is causing so much trouble. He says that inhaling nitrous oxide is common in local clubs and pubs, where it is sold openly for £2 per balloon as a variation on the 'lager and a shot' theme. He describes how it induces a brief 20- to 30-second period of elation with no real after-effects. He enjoyed the experience so much that he bought a carton of canisters online for his personal use. However, at the concert he was pressured by other students to share them and he sold a few for £2 – the same as in pubs.

An internet search carried out by a member of staff reveals that inhaling nitrous oxide is indeed common at certain clubs and rave parties, but it may not be as safe as it seems, with one death attributed to a combination of nitrous oxide, alcohol and other drugs. Strictly speaking, it is not illegal to purchase or sell small cannisters of nitrous oxide, but to buy them requires a declaration stating that the product is to be used in catering (for coffee frothing machines) and not for human consumption. Selling the drug for human use breaches the Medicines Act 1968[5] – this applies to all health professionals, including senior medical students. TW says that he was unaware of the seriousness of the behaviour – all he was doing was 'having a bit of fun in his own time', which had 'nothing to do with training to be a doctor'.

The case is referred to the Health and Conduct Committee for consideration, and then to the University Fitness to Practise Committee. By the time of the fitness to practise meeting 2 weeks later, the case is a common topic of conversation across the campus and in medical schools throughout the country. A local newspaper even runs a sensationalised story with the headline 'would you want this drug trafficker to be your doctor?' The committee is split between those who feel that this is silly behaviour by a young man that hurt no one and results in him learning a valuable lesson, and those who feel that a senior medical student (age 23) should know better and that selling the drug to others is a very serious matter. The university also informally consults the General Medical Council, which informs them that upon graduation the student would probably be formally investigated (i.e. prior to registration). After much discussion, the committee decides to expel TW. He appeals to the University Appeals Committee, but the decision is upheld.

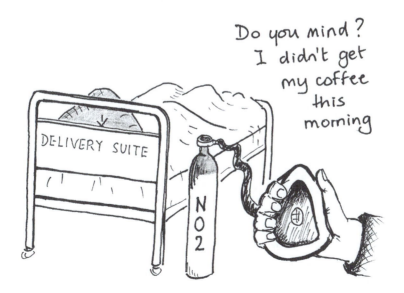

Questions

- (When) Should lack of maturity from a medical student be considered 'mitigation' when demonstrating unprofessional behaviour?
- To what extent should medical students be treated the same as registered doctors?
- Is it likely that the behaviour was judged differently because of publicity that accrued and concern for the university's reputation?
- The student had almost completed a medical degree before his expulsion, and now will probably find it difficult to gain a place at another school. Is this a case of 'a waste of talent' or of 'saving the public from danger in the nick of time'?
- Was the decision in this case too harsh, and was there an alternative course of action?

Discussion

This case could have arisen anywhere, and if this type of behaviour is indeed commonplace, it certainly gives cause for concern. Possibly, the element of selling in public was what called down the wrath of the university. Additionally, a punitive decision sets a powerful example to others. However, given the amount of attention this case received, the university should be careful not to expose students to 'trial by media'. This case may be more about damage control than individual justice or matters of patient safety. Because the case attracted so much attention, it was perhaps difficult for members of the school to act dispassionately, in much the same way that a crime committed in a very public way limits options for a fair trial; a jury (or members of a panel) may find it difficult to insulate itself from the outside 'noise'. It is notable that there was a split opinion on the panel in this case, indicating that members may have been conscious of dangers inherent in this situation.

It is important to form an objective judgement based on the facts of the case in isolation from the wider public debate. Deciding how to deal with a particular case requires a different mindset than that required for debating matters of public policy. It would be wrong to elide the two as if they were part of the same process; limiting the damage to an institution must be separate from the demands of justice, and in this case, TW's legal advisors could well have advocated challenging the expulsion and taking the university to court. Some people might argue that TW's mistake was 'getting caught', but that would be to condone inappropriate behaviours, especially with regard to a soon-to-be practising medical professional. Unprofessional behaviour is just that, particularly when it involves breaking a law designed to protect the public; ultimately each case can only be judged on its merits.

The next point to consider is whether and when it is appropriate to make allowances or show tolerance in light of someone's lack of maturity. Students aspiring to become practising health professionals should expect to be judged against the same standard as a health professional, but things are not always black and white. While it may seem reasonable to apply professional standards with regard to both the degree of risk posed to the public and the responsibility towards the care of patients at a given point in time during medical school, a final-year medical student may be held to a higher standard than a first-year undergraduate. TW certainly behaved inappropriately, but his behaviour falls more easily into the 'stupid and irresponsible' category than anything that implies criminal intent (acknowledging that there was a breach in the law).

The school may well have reacted overly harshly in their expulsion of TW, given that students who commit more serious offences are sometimes given further opportunities to prove themselves and remedy their behaviour. While TW did not behave well, the extent to which he posed a risk to the public is probably lower than in some other cases, and the regulator is best placed to form a judgement from a public safety perspective; the school could have chosen to leave it to the GMC to reach a decision on TW's future. The risks in pursuing this strategy are mainly reputational, as the school could *appear* to be in the wrong for allowing a student to graduate after such a public incident. If this student otherwise had a clean record, he could arguably be given a chance to complete his education, given the existence of a safety mechanism built in prior to his registration.

Summary

- In terms of professionalism, the school took the view that it was not possible to remediate TW's behaviour; however, professionalism issues need to be judged on their merits.
- The outcome was such that the interests of justice may not have been well served by an overly harsh judgement on a student in order to defend the university against a tide of public opinion.
- Patient safety is always an issue and public protection has to be borne in mind, but there is no clear evidence that allowing this student to graduate would compromise public safety (e.g. after passing some additional hurdles).
- Education and training were not central to this case.
- There is no suggestion that protocol was an issue; however, had the decision been challenged in court, the case could have ended differently.
- The regulator is aware of the inherent dangers in allowing a student to graduate with this type of behaviour on the record; the school was right to seek advice from the regulator but the university seemed to prejudge

the case by not allowing the regulator to review the case immediately post graduation.
- It is not possible to produce guidelines to cover every eventuality, but good guidelines should make it easier for a school or university to do its job.

CASE 3
A junior doctor serves prison time for being in possession of drugs.

Outline

Immediately following the breakdown of a personal relationship, RP, a first-year Foundation doctor, knows that he is not functioning well, but for various reasons he does not want to take time off. A few months after the split with his girlfriend, he is caught in possession of cannabis, a class C drug; he is required to pay a fine and receives a custodial sentence of 4 weeks in prison. As a consequence of this incident he is automatically referred to the General Medical Council (GMC). Following a fitness to practise hearing, he is suspended from the medical register for a period of 12 months.

RP fully accepts that he was in the wrong, but he tells a friend and colleague that he thinks he is being treated harshly. He does not think he was ever a risk to the public, and in his mind, he has never caused harm to anyone else. Furthermore, he recently heard about a case of a junior doctor who regularly smoked marijuana while having sexual relations with a patient, and while this doctor was struck off the register he did not go to jail. While RP was suspended rather than erased from the register by the GMC, he thinks that his own behaviour was less reprehensible. The other doctor, who was married and having intercourse with a vulnerable patient, and one who had a history of depression, in his view, had committed the greater 'crime'.

In order for RP to be able to stand a chance of resuming his career he has to try to keep his knowledge and skills up to date and engage with the deanery's rehabilitation programme. In a one-on-one session with a senior clinician, RP admits to having had '3 months of madness'. Furthermore, he knows that in order to stand a chance of being taken back on the register and re-employed he has to be totally honest. He owns up to the fact that he had experimented with drugs while at medical school, and in his first year had come before a disciplinary panel at the university. He and two of his friends had been caught 'doing soft drugs' at a music festival. At the time, the central university thought that there was no significant risk of bringing the school (or the medical profession) into disrepute, and he was allowed to continue on the programme with a written warning.

When RP applied for provisional registration with the GMC, prior to beginning Foundation training, he had to self-declare whether he had ever been before a disciplinary panel. Because a formal warning would have been in his student file, he put this down and the GMC then follows it up with the university. Since at that point it was perhaps a case of him being 'young and foolish', the GMC decided that there was no need to investigate the incident. However, when later convicted for the drug offence, the previous incident is seen in a different light, and now besides showing insight and remorse into his recent behaviour, he has to try to prove that this is not a weakness in his character. Academically, he always did well at medical school, with exam results that put him in the top quintile.

At this point, the deanery has the task of advising him on when or if to apply for reinstatement on the register. The combination of a police conviction, time spent in jail and the earlier incident at medical school does not look good. He needs to go to some lengths to stand a chance of being able to demonstrate that his behaviour is reformed and that there is no real likelihood of him reoffending. At the reinstatement hearing, which takes place towards the end of the period of suspension, he produces written testimony of good character and certificates of attendance for continuing medical education; RP informs the panel that he recently got married and that he now has a stable life. He is extremely remorseful and has insight into his previous poor behaviour. He no longer frets about having been treated harshly and is keen to get back to work as a practising clinician. The GMC panel decides to allow him to resume training under close supervision and with regular monitoring through the deanery.*

Questions
- How appropriate was the management of the case during medical school?
- In the absence of evidence of poor academic and clinical performance, how should drug use be managed?
- How feasible is the monitoring of drug use in the workplace?

Discussion
This case is primarily about drug use and poor judgement balanced against underlying intelligence and insight. Most medical schools and training programmes will have encountered similar cases, albeit with different twists and turns, but this does not make them easy to deal with. Everything hinges on the detail, and the facts rarely come to light all at once. When facts are revealed in a piecemeal fashion it can make a case easy to judge in hindsight but not so easy to deal with as it unfolds.

---

* A deanery is a local unit of organisation within the National Health Service for postgraduate medical education.

RP cannot escape the consequences of his past indiscretions, and the ultimate decision of the regulator may seem surprising; however, what probably tipped the balance in his favour was his willingness to come clean and disclose everything that needed to be out in the open. Without such transparency this case would certainly have spelt the end of RP's medical career. Clearly, he should have sought help when he was going through a difficult time as a junior doctor, but few people have the inclination or insight to seek out professional help when it is most needed. His ability to cope with emotional stress, however, may be limited, which is something he will have to come to terms with if he wants to avoid difficulties later on. While this could be seen as a character flaw, it is important to consider fairness and alternative courses of action.

Given that RP met all the requirements that were put to him by members of the GMC panel and that by this stage he was being honest and open, it might have been difficult to defend a harsher treatment, such as an extended period of suspension. One sometimes hears that nurses come out of this type of situation worse than doctors, and that medical regulators bend over backwards to look after 'one of their own'. However, such hearsay is difficult to justify,[6] and the lay contribution to GMC adjudication processes should help to guard against such allegations of protectionism.[7] It is not the case that senior clinicians are allowed to judge their juniors behind closed doors; at least one member of the panel will be non-medical. Furthermore, everything will become a matter of public record (unless the case is dismissed as being without foundation and having no penalty).

Public interest is often best served by giving a well-trained doctor a second chance to prove him- or herself, unless the doctor presents a real danger to the public or to patients. Panellists have to take this into consideration and strike a balance between listening to the needs of doctors and listening to the needs of patients who might be in their care. Fairness and transparency are key here.

Summary

- Within this case we see elements of professionalism and unprofessionalism, and RP's response to the latter enabled him to demonstrate aspects of the former. His belated insight does not right previous wrongs, but it mitigates to the extent that it allows those adjudicating to consider alternative courses of action.
- One's emotional reaction to a case such as this should not lead one to a premature judgement; different elements of the case have to be weighed one against another. There is no evidence that the doctor was treated unfairly; the panel in the final hearing may have been taking a risk, but it was a calculated one prefaced by an overt demonstration of changed attitudes and behaviours.

- Public protection was a critical element in this case and it would be inconceivable for RP to have been allowed to continue practising after receiving a custodial sentence; however, circumstances do not always remain the same, and had he been denied the chance to go back to work, RP's earlier premonition of having been unfairly treated might have proved correct.
- There may be little that can be done through education to prevent such a case; human nature is frail and people do bad things, whether they are educated or not. Medical educators have to deal with such cases, and this case serves to highlight a need for educators to develop necessary skills to be able to confront difficult tasks.
- Protocol was followed in this case and the procedures already in place proved their worth.
- It is easy to criticise a public body because you do not like a particular decision, but regulation probably worked well in this case; it is hard to satisfy public expectation while maintaining good relations with the public, the profession and government.
- This case does not raise any issues with regard to guidelines.

CASE 4

A trainee who is under pressure is found self-prescribing.

Outline

RD is a second-year resident in the anaesthesiology residency training programme. Her internship year in internal medicine was spent at another academic medical centre and she came highly recommended to this programme, starting in postgraduate year 2. Her first 3 months in the programme are unremarkable, other than her tendency to be late in the morning. She is well liked among her peers and appropriately apologetic when she is late. Halfway through her first year in the programme, RD starts to lose significant amounts of weight. Her peers notice a marked shift in her mood. There are rumours about an illness in her family, but her performance has not suffered and, out of respect for her privacy, her programme director does not ask any questions about her personal life. During her fourth month in the programme she calls in sick for 3 days, and on the fourth day she submits a written request for a medical leave of absence, accompanied by a psychiatrist's note indicating that a 2-month leave of absence will be necessary for medical reasons. The programme director grants RD's leave request, and then grants a 1-month extension, in accordance with institutional policy.

At the end of this extended period of paid leave, RD returns to work with a medical clearance letter signed by the same physician who had signed the initial letter advising the need for leave. Upon her return, supervisors and peers immediately note RD's erratic performance. She is frequently tearful and her lateness is chronic. She has lost more weight and she seems frail compared with how she used to appear. After just 2 weeks, her programme director is concerned and invites RD to meet and discuss whether she is well enough to be at work. She explains that when she first requested leave, her 30-year-old husband had been diagnosed with a terminal illness and she became clinically depressed. Since then, her husband had died and she had been admitted for inpatient psychiatric treatment. She is continuing in outpatient therapy and after the 3 months away, she had thought she was ready to return to work. Now she realises that she needs some more time. The programme director is sympathetic to RD's tragic situation and grants 1 month's personal unpaid leave.

One week into this period, the programme director receives an alarming call from a local pharmacist. The pharmacist called to report an unusual prescribing pattern linked to the prescription pad issued to RD as a member of the training programme. Further investigation reveals that RD has been writing and/or calling in numerous prescriptions for controlled substances, allegedly for her sister, during the entire period of leave. The programme director immediately calls RD's home and has difficulty reaching her. After numerous phone messages and a certified letter, he eventually succeeds in getting a response and RD agrees to a meeting.

RD admits that her leaves of absence are not only related to grief and clinical depression but also to prescription drug addiction, for which she would be seeking further inpatient treatment. She confesses to having called in and written the narcotics prescriptions for personal use/abuse. Tearfully, RD explains that her downward spiral over the past few months is linked to her husband's untimely death and that she is confident that, with treatment, she should recover and be able to return to training. RD asks the programme director to show understanding for her plight as a patient as well as a resident. She says that it is critical to her recovery for her to be permitted to resign and to get her life back on track without any disciplinary action or notification to the state. She explains that she still wants to pursue her lifelong ambition of becoming a physician. The programme director concludes the meeting and lets RD know that she will be hearing from him soon.

After consultation with legal counsel for the hospital, the programme director informs RD that the programme would accept her resignation, but that the institution will be obligated to report the resignation in lieu of disciplinary action. Alternatively, the programme would suspend and dismiss RD from the programme; however, she would be entitled to an appeal. The programme director explains to RD that he and the institution could not violate their legal and ethical obligations regarding her training and potential future as a physician.

Questions

- How common is it for supervisors and co-residents to ignore signs that a resident's lateness or change in behaviour may be related to psychiatric illness or substance abuse?
- Should a programme director ask questions about a trainee's health beyond what is written in a 'doctor's note' requesting medical leave?
- The programme director must balance concern for the trainee's health and well-being with issues of patient safety; what type of professional help could or should have been offered early on, and where is the line between someone's personal and professional life drawn?
- What are the programme director's obligations as regards terminating RD's training and reporting to the state licensing authority?

Discussion

Initially, the challenge in RD's case stemmed from the fact that, while her behaviour and appearance changed, her performance was consistent. Because she was a very private person, her co-residents and programme director were not aware of her husband's illness and her extreme distress and depression. To her credit, RD sought medical help and took a medical leave before her impairment affected patient care or became evident to peers or supervisors. More often, trainees suffering from psychiatric or substance abuse issues lack the awareness that their behaviour may pose a risk to themselves and to patient safety. Nonetheless, RD's eagerness to return to training coupled with her need to continue to receive a pay cheque drove her to return prematurely. This experience highlights the need to consider carefully a trainee's fitness, even upon receipt of medical clearance to return to work after a leave of absence. Programme directors must rely on supervising physicians and co-trainees to report any concerning behaviour in the interests of the trainee and the over-riding obligation to protect patient safety.

Sadly, RD's behaviour while on leave gave the programme director little opportunity to help her as a trainee. The programme director was extremely sympathetic to her situation and wanted to do all he could to support her recovery efforts. However, once it was established that she had fraudulently written prescriptions using the programme's identifier, she could not be accepted back into the programme, and the reporting obligation could not be avoided.

Summary

- RD's substance abuse and psychiatric issues linked with poor judgement caused her to violate the law. The most significant lapse in professionalism was her decision to write prescriptions for herself in her sister's name using the programme's prescription pad.

- We believe that the outcome was fair and appropriate, although the situation was equally distressing to her supervisors and co-residents.
- Because RD was not working for most of the time she was impaired, there was no patient harm. However, if the programme director had not taken the appropriate actions, patients could have been put at risk.
- Programme directors and fellow trainees need to be alert to erratic behaviour; supervisors and programme directors are encouraged to be attuned to their residents and to recommend counselling or other forms of support.
- In spite of the personal desire to give her a second chance, there was no alternative to making a report to the state licensing board.
- The pharmacist notified relevant authorities regarding fraudulent prescriptions, and once notified, a state licensing board has to act.
- The definition of professional misconduct under state law was considered. RD violated state law regarding prescription writing.

CASE 5

A medical student is arrested and faces drugs charges.

Outline

The dean of students receives a call from campus police to alert her that the city police department has arrested a second-year medical student, DA. DA is charged with leading a criminal conspiracy to distribute illicit substances, including pain medications and amphetamines that are often prescribed for attention deficit disorder. The dean of students warns members of her staff to expect to see this reported in the local press. She contacts legal counsel to find out how to contact DA, who remains in police custody; the advice received is to send a message of support. In addition, counsel advises her to warn members of faculty not to contact DA, which could require them to testify about their conversations in court.

The dean of students notifies the chair of the Medical Student Progress Committee (MSPC) and gives a full account of the story to the committee at the next meeting. By this stage, DA has already been released on bail; the dean of students and the student's academic advisor then meet with DA and express their support but tell him explicitly that it is not in his interest to discuss details of the charges with either of them. DA's student record shows no previous incidents of unprofessional behaviour. The MSPC has no independent method to determine what took place, having not conducted its own investigations.

However, taking into account the allegation of engaging in behaviour that would directly harm others and the criminal charges that the student is facing (covered by the school's policy on professionalism), the committee votes to place him on administrative leave, thus prohibiting him from attending all classes.

DA tries to access the university health resources as he feels he would benefit from therapy to help him cope with the stress of his current circumstances. He could talk things over while still being protected from disclosure in court by reason of confidentiality within the doctor–patient relationship. He books treatment, but because of his current status the cost of treatment is only partly covered by DA's health plan, which somewhat adds to his worries.

The dean continues to offer support to DA on a regular basis, and both parties agree not to discuss anything related to the legal proceedings. The student expects to be placed on trial within 6 months, and he's eventually found guilty on most of the charges (including several felony charges, which are the most serious level of charges under the US justice system). Despite this being his first offence, DA is sentenced to 4 years' imprisonment. At its next meeting the MSPC discusses the findings of the jury, and it votes to dismiss him from medical school because of his unprofessional behaviour. DA does not appeal the decision.

Questions
- What is the role of a medical school during a criminal investigation and trial of one of its students?
- Was the school correct in putting DA on administrative leave when it did?
- How should the MSPC go about making a determination on activities that took place outside the school? Can it justify the outcome if as a result of the process, the student is disqualified and prevented from continuing on the course?

Discussion
Unprofessional behaviour that occurs outside the medical setting reflects on the reputation of the individual student, on the institution itself and on the profession as a whole. Reports of unprofessional behaviour outside the medical setting are often difficult to contextualise, and their relevance in terms of professionalism is difficult to determine; however, when a report is deemed to be accurate, and when behaviours are consistent with difficulties that a student has in professional settings, then such reports have their value. At times, the unprofessional behaviour exhibited by a trainee outside of a medical setting is so egregious that it alone can be cause for a review of a trainee's fitness for a career as a physician. This case illustrates this concept well, as the student

is engaged in a pattern of behaviour that is directly linked to harming others through the distribution of illegal substances; in this case there is little room for moral ambiguity. The school cannot interfere with a criminal investigation and can only provide evidence when asked.

This case emphasises the importance of involving legal counsel early and often in the process of determining how to evaluate and manage a student's unprofessional behaviour. In this instance, the dean of students receives important legal advice about potential risks to both the student and the dean if she converses with DA about details surrounding his arrest. This prohibition complicates the work of the MSPC, as the dean of students and members of the committee are not able to collect data pertinent to developing an institutional response. Under the law, the student is presumed innocent until found guilty; however, it would be highly imprudent for the MSPC to allow a student charged with very serious unprofessional and potentially illegal behaviour to continue in the role of a medical professional trainee.

The MSPC eventually reaches the conclusion that since legal proceedings evaluated the evidence of illegal behaviour, and with the aid of a jury, it found DA guilty beyond reasonable doubt, then the committee has to rely on the court's judgement in terms of assessing the professionalism. A criminal conviction of this nature is by definition unprofessional, and the committee has no real alternative but to vote to dismiss the student. However, if DA had already been a fully qualified medical practitioner, there would have been some additional steps to be taken.

Summary
- Behaviour that occurs outside the medical setting can still be considered unprofessional. While in this case the behaviours were not independently assessed, it is clear that a criminal conviction of this kind makes it effectively impossible for DA to be allowed to continue his medical training.
- Physicians in training should never engage in behaviours that could seriously harm others; in this case, the behaviour was clearly illegal as well as unprofessional, and so the outcome seems fair and proportionate.
- Patient safety and public protection considerations would have been part of the thinking behind the MSPC's decision; the committee has a moral and legal duty to help safeguard others.
- Training and education may not be sufficient to eliminate the possibility of someone committing gross professional misconduct. Regrettably, doctors and medical students occasionally commit serious crimes.
- While legal protocol constrained what the dean of students and MSPC were able to do, there was no question of a systems failure.

- When serious legal implications arise in relation to a medical student or trainee's behaviour, it is advisable for senior members of the school to consult legal counsel early and often. However, it is important to remember that conversations between physicians and trainees are not protected from disclosure in legal proceedings in the same way that they are between doctor and patient. Since the case is about a medical student who is eventually dismissed, the regulator plays no part.
- Guidelines were not utilised in this case.

CASE 6

A trainee with a pattern of poor attendance attributes this to his sick dog.

Outline

A first-year psychiatry resident, PW, is brought to the attention of the programme director; hospital staff where the resident works are worried as he has not shown up for work and he has not been in touch with his supervisor. The supervisor tries to call him but PW does not respond to his pager or his phone. The programme director tries to call but also receives no response. The next day PW turns up for work saying that a family member in an adjoining state has become ill and that he has been called in to help. He explains how he left in a rush and forgot his pager and phone, and he forgot to call his supervisor. The programme director admonishes him about attending to his professional responsibilities but accepts the explanation.

A few months later the programme director receives a call from the resident claiming that he's being treated unfairly. Staff at the hospital are upset because on several occasions PW called in to say that he wouldn't be in for work. He says he was unable to work because his pet dog became comatose, and the veterinarian had suggested taking the dog to a veterinary hospital 4 hours' drive away, because there they have specialised facilities for managing such disorders. PW called in to his supervisors, as he had been advised, but feels that the supervisors and co-residents are not understanding of his situation. He recently moved to the city and has no friends or colleagues to help him manage the dog.

The programme director calls the supervising physician at the hospital, who states that PW has been away from work three times in the past 2 weeks because of the dog's illness. The supervisor goes on to say that co-residents are upset with PW, not only because they have to cover his work but also because they feel that when he signs out at the end of a shift, he has not properly completed his work before leaving. The programme director asks the supervising physician whether she has discussed any of this with the resident; she answers no, saying that the programme director recently emphasised how Accreditation Council for Graduate Medical Education duty hour rules mandate that residents must leave at the end of 16 hours of duty in the hospital. While PW is slow in completing his assignments he does not appear to be purposefully shirking his patient care activities.

The programme director travels to the hospital to meet with the resident so PW does not again have to leave the hospital in order to attend the meeting. PW doesn't show up at the agreed time, and once again he does not respond to his pager or phone. The programme director travels back, and staff at the office continue the attempts to try to reach him. When they do eventually succeed, PW states that he was in the cafeteria, which is where he had been told to go by the programme director's assistant. Unfortunately, the assistant had put the wrong meeting place in the calendar, and she also gave out wrong information when the programme director rang to confirm details. PW apologises for not having his phone or pager on him (again), this time saying that he was running late and in haste had forgotten to pick up the pager and phone. In the context of a range of other issues that had been brought to his attention, the programme director finds his patience beginning to wane, even though this time the error is partly attributable to his assistant.

PW meets with the programme director the next day and says that his dog's health has improved and that he does not think he will need to have to take any further time off. He denies signing off work more often than other residents and apologises profusely for the business of forgetting his pager and phone. The programme director emphasises the importance of PW being scrupulous in his communications with co-residents and supervisors (and remembering to bring his pager and phone to work) if PW is to regain his colleagues' trust. The programme director also asks whether PW thanked colleagues who had covered for him during his absence; it turns out that he had not but pledges that he will do so as soon as possible.

The programme director discusses the 'slippery slope' of professionalism, noting that when there is a pattern of unprofessional behaviours and absences and a new concern arises, it is likely to be seen as another example of unprofessional behaviour rather than just an innocent oversight. He gives the example of his own experience when PW did not show up for their meeting, and how because of the previous issues he at first assumed that the resident was at fault.

At the next meeting of the Resident Progress Committee (RPC) (comprising faculty representing each of the institutions and a resident from each year of the programme), the programme director presents his findings. Review of evaluations from nursing staff also note concerns about PW not responding promptly to pages. The committee agrees that PW seems to be struggling with professionalism but that this should be seen in the context of his being a first-year resident. The committee agrees that the programme director should write a letter to PW expressing the concerns of the RPC about the importance of developing better professional behaviours. They assign a mentor to PW to discuss issues relating to professionalism. The chief resident, whose position is to serve as a liaison between faculty and residents, volunteers to take on this role.

He agrees to meet with PW on a weekly basis over breakfast. The chief also talks with supervising faculty to gather feedback on how well PW is managing his professional responsibilities, listening for any concerns that may be raised by co-residents. The chief talks with PW about strategies for managing day-to-day professional challenges and improving efficiency in completing patient care activities. PW is diligent about following up on these suggestions and brings along some good questions relating to professionalism and supervision. One example of an attempt to repair relationships with his colleagues was to sponsor a party at his house where he introduces colleagues to his dog over supper and provides homemade food, plus drinks and a movie.

By the end of the year the chief resident reports to the RPC that PW seems to have made good adjustments to managing his professional responsibilities, commenting that in part, this is due to his organising several social outings and becoming a popular member of the residency class. In his end-of-year meeting with the programme director, PW reports how he feels much more confident now and that he has a better understanding of the need to maintain his professional responsibilities. At its next meeting the RPC votes to send a letter to PW congratulating him on successfully remediating concerns that the committee had regarding his previous lack of professionalism; no further complaints arise during the rest of his residency.

Questions

- To what do you attribute PW's successful remediation? Were the interventions successful, and, if so, why?
- What lessons does this case provide in terms of monitoring trainees?
- What value should a programme place on encouraging social interaction among trainees?

Discussion

This case illustrates how trainees with professionalism challenges can be successfully remediated. In the authors' experience, this is best accomplished when problem behaviours are dealt with as and when they occur, and when they are clearly identified early on as being about professionalism. Problems that remain unresolved often affect others, and they can significantly affect a trainee's future career; assigning a mentor is one way of helping residents with their professional behaviours. However, each of these steps can be challenging for education leaders to accomplish. Supervisors are often quite good at verbally talking about professionalism problems with one another and with programme directors, but they do not always address these issues directly with the trainee or write the problems up in evaluations. Such responses are not helpful, and a further problem is that unprofessional behaviours may first present with peers or in interactions with other disciplines such as nursing (i.e. not with the supervisor). In this case, supervisors may be unaware of what is happening until matters are brought to their attention. If done well, the use of multirater evaluations (completed by peers and allied health disciplines) can provide good opportunities for collecting data from various sources.

Early career trainees may see professionalism as a concept that is pertinent only to their interactions with patients and their families. They may not fully understand their professional responsibilities to colleagues, institutions and to the community, as in this case, where the resident did not know about his behaviour affecting colleagues or that it raised issues of professionalism. The conversation with the programme director proved helpful; discussion about the slippery slope of unprofessional behaviours and the need to establish and maintain the trust of colleagues can help motivate trainees to work on some of these problems.

Committees addressing trainee deficiencies in professionalism can struggle to develop effective plans to remediate poor behaviour. A letter that clearly defines the behaviours that are considered unprofessional, stating that the behaviours must change, can be a helpful intervention. In such a case, the letter may note how it is the trainee's responsibility to try to change these behaviours. Appointing a senior colleague in the role of special supervisor underscores the importance that the committee places on the need to improve behaviours, providing a role model figure who is able to develop strategies and monitor their implementation. A senior resident with good professional skills can be especially effective, since the power relationship between senior and junior residents can allow a resident to be more forthcoming about challenges faced than might otherwise be the case (e.g. with a senior member of academic faculty).

Summary
- Maintaining collegial relationships with colleagues and supervisors was the main professionalism issue in this case, and these issues seem to have been properly addressed.
- The outcome appears fair and just.
- Patient safety and public protection were not significant issues in this case, even though it can only be a question of time before unresolved professionalism issues directly affect patients, especially when a resident is absent on multiple occasions.

- The importance of maintaining good collegial relations has implications in terms of designing effective education and training programmes.
- Protocol was not an issue in this case.
- Neither were there any issues that need concern the regulator.
- National guidelines recommend reviewing each resident competency every 6 months; while duty hours are a matter of local concern, poor attendance clearly has wider professionalism implications.

CASE 7
A 'successful' trainee has poor interactions with colleagues, most of them female.

Outline
KP, a second-year female internal medicine resident, graduated from medical school in Russia and is repeatedly brought to the attention of the programme director because of alleged unprofessional interactions with supervisors, junior residents and nursing staff. The programme director had not previously experienced any issues with her; in fact, he thinks she is one of the best residents in the programme in terms of her fund of knowledge and technical skills such as central line placement. He also knows that senior clinicians in the subspecialty she is likely to enter (cardiology) also think highly of her. However, complaints come from colleagues whom he respects, from junior residents he knows to be straightforward, and from senior nursing staff with significant previous experience.

The programme director's preliminary investigations show that professionalism complaints centre on several issues. The supervisors who have difficulty with her say she does not follow advice, and sometimes she neglects patients under her care. Junior residents report that KP is unrelentingly critical of them and never helps them to complete tasks or teach them procedures; finally, nurses report that she is aloof and condescending in her interactions with them. The programme director finds she scores very highly on the yearly examination of knowledge in internal medicine and that her reviews are at the extremes – either very positive or very negative. Interestingly, as the programme director investigates these claims, he notes that individuals having difficulties with KP are almost entirely women. In discussions with KP, the programme director is struck by her sense that senior clinicians, junior residents and nurses all seem jealous of her success in the specialty. KP explains how she feels that she gets bad reviews because colleagues do not want to see a particularly attractive young woman succeed in the specialty, and especially so in that she graduated overseas.

Because of repeated and serious complaints about her professional behaviour (including not responding to instructions from attending physicians), the programme director decides to bring this to the attention of the Resident Progress Committee (RPC). The RPC suggests that the resident should be counselled about perceptions that others have of her, and the committee provides her with a mentor to talk about whether her behaviour with female health professionals can be changed. A senior female physician in the department, who went to medical school in Eastern Europe, agrees to serve as a mentor to KP. They begin to meet on a weekly basis to discuss KP's style of interacting with other physicians, trainees and staff. They schedule a total of six sessions over 2 months; however, KP states that her schedule in the medical intensive care unit (MICU) is such that she will be unable to continue with the appointments. During this time, KP has two good rotation reviews with male physicians; however, she has a poor review from the female physician supervising the MICU rotation. The review speaks of technical failings to do with test values that the senior physician thinks are critical; furthermore, KP fails to evaluate a patient whom the supervisor told her to prioritise. Poor reviews from junior residents continue to be received, and several new written complaints come in from nursing staff in MICU.

The programme director again meets with KP to review the evaluations and her decision not to utilise the mentor that the programme director has assigned to her. KP says she thinks that reports from the attending physician are inaccurate, and she forcefully expresses the opinion that when male residents display similar behaviours the behaviours are considered perfectly normal. The programme director passes these comments on to the committee chair, but when the RPC meets, it votes to place the resident on probation, informing her that if her professional behaviours do not improve she could be dismissed from the programme.

In her next rotation, the programme director receives two additional complaints from female physicians claiming that the resident is dismissive of their instructions; in addition, another complaint is received from a junior resident. After these findings are received, the RPC votes to dismiss the resident. In a meeting with the programme director to discuss the decision, KP is informed of her right to appeal. She asks to appeal the RPC decision to the chair of the department, and KP is placed on paid administrative leave while the review is being conducted.

The department chair appoints a senior male faculty member to conduct a review of the case; he reviews each of the letters the programme director wrote to the resident after meetings of the RPC, and he meets with several faculty members as well as with KP. He notes the allegation of gender bias and tries to assess whether any of the accusations made against her are unfair. In his report to the chair, the senior faculty member determines that the process developed by the programme director was fair and allowed for due process. However, he notes that extenuating circumstances contributed to one or two individual incidents, and in those instances, in his opinion, KP provided an acceptable standard of care. He also notes that while he has been unable to find evidence of a clear gender bias against KP, female faculty members and nurses managed to develop positive mentoring relationships with other female residents in the department. Furthermore, he sees that complaints from junior residents come from both men and women.

In his report, he recommends that the RPC should meet again, and after reading this review, the committee again reaches a decision to dismiss the resident. As before, KP appeals this decision to the chair; when he upholds the committee's decision she exerts her right to appeal to the chief of staff at the hospital. The chief of staff convenes a panel of three senior clinicians, comprising two women and one man; it conducts a review of all the documentation, including the report of the senior faculty members, interviewing KP and several faculty members. After 4 months of investigation, the panel concludes that due process has been followed, and the chief of staff writes to the chair of the department, who informs KP that she must leave the programme. No further opportunities are left for her to appeal.

Questions
- How should a training programme assess allegations of gender bias, and to what extent is gender bias the main issue?
- Complaints were received from a variety of sources, and the process of investigation was necessarily complex; how easy is it to cut through the fog and reach a clear, defensible conclusion on the most appropriate outcome for a case such as this?

Discussion
This case raises important issues to consider when allegations of unprofessional behaviour arise. Bias in the evaluation process caused by race, ethnicity, gender, age and sexual orientation (depending on institutional and government policy) are prohibited by law, and allegations of bias inevitably give rise to questions of due process. Determining whether a group of faculty members are biased against a trainee can be more challenging than when allegations are directed at a single supervisor, and in this case, the allegation of gender discrimination is made against same-sex members of the faculty as well as hospital staff. This does not change the seriousness of the allegation, requiring senior staff to undertake the formal process of review. Careful attention to the composition of the RPC and appeal committees is required so as to ensure that they are sufficiently representative.

For cultural reasons, unprofessional behaviours that occur with residents who did their primary medical training in another country can lead to special challenges. The Accreditation Council for Graduate Medical Education regulations require that residents be taught about American culture and about the culture of medicine, stating that:

> Fellows must demonstrate competence in their knowledge of American culture and subcultures, including immigrant populations, particularly those found in the patient community associated with the educational program, with specific focus on the cultural elements of the relationship between the fellow and the patient including the dynamics of differences in cultural identity, values and preferences, and power.[8]

However, these requirements are often difficult to implement. In this case, appointing a mentor with similar experiences in terms of prior training should help in developing a useful relationship in which a resident's difficulties can be discussed in a simple, straightforward manner. When a resident's continued participation in a programme is at risk, providing time for these sessions is something that should be actively encouraged.

The standard for a fair review process requires a written protocol, including a proper process for appeals. Documentation of communications between education leaders and the resident is a critical component of the process. This documentation is best developed with input from senior institutional leadership (such as a director of graduate medical education and/or institutional legal counsel). Documentation should make clear what remediation plans were put forward, and what evidence and timeframes were utilised when determining whether or not a trainee successfully remediated the difficulties that had been identified.

In this instance, the appeals process finds that data reviewed by the RPC was not fully accurate, which raises questions as to whether the committee could continue to be involved with adjudicating the case. Multiple levels of appeal help to ensure fair process, enabling a committee to assess thoroughly the allegations of unprofessional behaviour. In this case, the appeal process took over 6 months to complete, and it is likely that a resident would continue to be paid throughout this process. Professionalism issues encountered by KP affected colleagues from different branches of the profession and at different levels of seniority. While the amount of institutional resources used to investigate a case such as this are considerable, the cost of failing to conduct a proper investigation are potentially far greater in terms of reputational damage to the school and to the profession.

Summary

- Investigations of unprofessional behaviour must carefully determine whether a behaviour was unprofessional or whether there were any extenuating circumstances; KP's case is complex, and complex cases are always difficult to judge.
- For a committee process to be credible it must be able to demonstrate ability to conduct a fair review. There are different elements to this case, some of which, it could be argued, are fairer than others.
- Patient safety and public protection are not major issues in this case.
- Institutions need to be sure that their processes and procedures can withstand close scrutiny, and they ought to be subject to periodic review.
- Review committees should strive to be representative in terms of gender, cultural or ethnic backgrounds and under-represented minorities. Appeal processes must be thorough and allow adequate opportunities for review, even if this means taking a long time.
- No issues for the regulator arise from this case, although quality assurance and validation processes should ensure that committee structure and appeals processes are fit for purpose.
- Equal opportunity law was a point of reference in this case, although no discrimination or gender bias was actually found proven.

CASE 8

A trainee wants to leave the programme mid-year, claiming he is homesick.

Outline

JD, a 25-year-old male paediatrics resident, is in the middle of his second year of residency when he schedules an appointment with the programme director. He explains at the meeting that he is homesick and wants to return home; he lives in another state. The programme director enquires about whether JD is satisfied with the programme, or whether there is a personal reason for him wanting to return home. The resident denies any problem with the programme, stating that so far he is enjoying the residency and would strongly encourage others to consider the programme for their training; it is simply a matter of being homesick.

The programme director reminds JD about professional obligations that he would be abrogating by leaving the residency programme mid-year. JD says he is aware that he has a contract for a full year but that he does not believe the programme would be significantly affected by his absence. The programme director reminds him of the effect his leaving could have on patient care; he asks JD what could be done to help him stay in order to complete the year, or at least to stay until someone is found who can take his place. For JD to leave suddenly would mean that patients who have already been assigned to him may not have a designated physician to care for them. JD responds by saying that he knows the programme has managed in the past to rearrange rotations and have trainees who are on elective periods step in to fill the gap. The programme director reminds him of the extra overnight calls that his colleagues would have to take, explaining that when this happened before there was an angry response from residents who had to work the extra shifts. JD says he has already considered this inconvenience, but since the programme is a large one, each resident would only have to work two extra shifts to make up for his absence.

Discussions go back and forth, and the programme director reminds him again that he is under contract and points out that abrogation of his contract could create legal liabilities that JD would be well advised to consider. The programme director asks JD to reflect on these issues, saying that if JD needs to take a short break and go home to sort out any difficulties, he would do his best to work with JD and accommodate this request. However, JD would need to fulfil his professional responsibilities until the end of the academic year. The resident replies, saying that he will consider the offer of a respite period at home but that he is fairly certain he will not change his mind. A further meeting is scheduled in 3 days' time.

In the interim period between the first and second meetings, the programme director hears from another resident that JD's father has become ill and requires additional care at home. However, the informant states that he does not want this information to be shared with the resident, as he was told of this in confidence. When the next meeting between JD and the programme director takes place, JD repeats that his reason for wanting to leave is homesickness. He reports having thought carefully about the points raised at the initial meeting, but he says that he is not convinced that a decision to leave would have a material effect on patient care and that his leaving would only have a minimal effect on co-residents.

JD wants to leave immediately after completing the current rotation; the programme director points out that when he applies for a licence or hospital privileges, the programme director will be asked to fill out a form or write a letter. He would be obliged to state the resident's method of leaving the programme and to state that JD had not behaved in a professional manner in leaving the way that he did. Leaving with so little notice will have a negative impact on patient care as well as on peers and colleagues. JD responds by saying he is sorry the programme director feels this way but that he believes his performance so far has been of high quality and that he has fulfilled professional responsibilities to his patients in an exemplary manner. Indeed, review of his end-of-rotation global assessment forms is notable for the finding that his supervisors rate him highly on each of his Accreditation Council for Graduate Medical Education (ACGME) general medical competencies, including professionalism.

JD is set to leave the programme after completing the current patient care rotation, which gives the programme director 3 weeks in which to develop and implement plans for coverage. Details of the situation are presented to the Resident Progress Committee (RPC) of the department, comprising both faculty and trainees. The RPC agrees that JD's behaviour is unprofessional and that it should be reported to licensing and hospital credentialing boards when they enquire about his training record in the future. After discussions with legal counsel, the department does not pursue any legal claims against the resident for breach of contract, and the programme director writes a report on JD's behaviour at the time of leaving, outlining all the facts. This information will become a permanent part of JD's record.*

When later asked to comment on the resident's professional behaviour for hospital privileges or licensure, the programme director rates JD with a below-average score for professionalism. When further inquiries are made by credentialing agencies, the programme director reports that this unprofessional behaviour occurred in the context of JD leaving the programme, but he notes that during the year and a half that the resident was in the programme his professional behaviour was not called into question. It is likely that JD will subsequently have to explain about his behaviour to regulators and hospital administrators; however, it is not known whether this actually caused a licensing board or hospital to fail to provide a licence or hospital privileges.

Questions

- Was JD correct in assuming that his absence would not directly affect patient care? What was the main breach of professionalism?
- Should legal action have been pursued against JD for breach of contract?
- Were the steps taken by the programme director sufficient to ensure that the process was equitable and fair?

Discussion

In the United States, residents occupy a unique position of being both students and employees; they enjoy the advantages of being an employee (receiving a salary and benefits) as well as those of being a student (having protected time for study and professional development). The ACGME requires that all residents have a signed employment contract with the institution sponsoring the

---

* In the United States, whenever a physician applies for a state licence or privileges at a hospital or health-care institution, each previous place of training or employment is contacted and asked to attest to the physician's level of ability against a range of different measures, including professional behaviour.

residency programme. These contracts are binding on both parties, although in practice the sponsoring institution is usually held more accountable than the resident when breaches occur. This was true in this case, and although the programme director suggests legal action could be taken against JD, no legal claim was actually pursued.

This case highlights the fact that trainees can demonstrate good professional behaviour and yet have one episode of highly unprofessional behaviour that follows them throughout their professional career. Prior to this episode JD had been a model resident, receiving high marks on each end-of-rotation ACGME general medical competency, including professionalism. The case raises an interesting question about the degree to which unprofessional behaviour is subjectively determined. For the programme director, JD leaving unexpectedly in the middle of a year is highly unprofessional behaviour, leaving patients without a doctor and requiring colleagues to cover his professional responsibilities. However, others might think differently, and this clearly includes JD. Leaving without a valid reason challenges the fundamental tenet of professionalism – namely, placing the needs of patients above one's own. From a resident's perspective, JD completed patient care responsibilities in the current rotation and left with sufficient time for the programme to invoke coverage plans (which were already in existence to provide coverage for absences due to illness or other types of leave), making it difficult to fully repudiate JD's position.

Given the power relationship that exists between a programme director and a resident, it is important to ensure that the senior's perspective is not automatically validated and that decisions need to be subjected to a process of review. Presentation of the case to the RPC and university legal counsel provided the means by which this case was reviewed, confirming that the programme director's perspective about JD's behaviour was supported by other members of the department, including residents, thereby ensuring that due process was available to the resident in question.

All of this could have been avoided had JD been receptive to advice and accepted the offer of being allowed time to go home, and returning in order to complete the year. This case involves a resident making a deliberate choice in full knowledge of the consequences, and one suspects that 'homesickness' was being used as a mask to conceal something more personal. While JD may live to regret this decision, at the time he did not seem to accept that he was acting unprofessionally. There was very little the programme director could do to steer him away from his chosen course of action.

Summary

- Placing personal interests above patient care is the overarching concern here in terms of professionalism. Taking care not to be burdening one's colleagues unreasonably (e.g. for non-emergency issues) is the most significant factor, although having regard for the burden placed on programme administrators is also relevant.

- The outcome seems fair in that the programme director followed due process by consulting others and warning JD about the risks associated with leaving early; what is not known is the long-term impact that this might have on JD's career.
- Having proper regard for the need to provide patient care is a patient safety or public protection issue; JD did not seem to be mindful of this, although it proved difficult to refute his argument that systems existed to cope with unexpected absences.
- Being professional means being mindful of one's professional responsibilities in all areas all of the time. In a situation such as this, a major lapse in professionalism follows one throughout an entire career.
- Power relationships should be tempered by involving a wide range of professional opinion (including other trainees) to guard against subjective interpretations of professionalism; involving legal counsel is also part of the protocol for resolving matters of this kind.
- Involving the regulators (i.e. state licensing agencies and hospital credentialing boards) is an important part of the process; without these checks problem behaviours could recur or go undetected until the point where significant harm is caused; regulators are routinely notified about significant problems through their contact with programme administrators.
- Guidelines were not utilised in this case.

CASE 9
A trainee has strong technical skills but a bad temper.

Outline

SN is a third-year resident in the plastic surgery training programme. Throughout his first 2 years of training SN consistently receives high praise for his surgical skill and fund of knowledge. However, some performance evaluations note his impatience with medical students and nursing staff. When the programme director reminds SN of the need to show respect to the entire team he seems to accept the feedback.

Halfway through his third year, SN assists in surgery on a young patient who unexpectedly has a poor outcome and dies. SN flies into a rage when he learns of this death. He shouts at the nursing staff on the post-operative unit, calling them stupid and slow. The next day, when he encounters the intern who had been covering the patient the night before, in front of patients and family members he angrily accuses her of killing his patient. Upon learning of SN's outbursts, the programme director calls him into his office and immediately institutes a remediation plan aimed at anger management and working on his professionalism. SN is warned that failure to improve his behaviour will otherwise result in probation and ultimately, dismissal. SN accepts the remediation plan and promises to reform his behaviour. However, in a lengthy email to the programme director, he claims that the coverage of this service is inadequate and he blames the patient death on inaccessibility of the fellow on call, the inexperience of the intern, and the incompetence of nursing staff.

He attends the mandatory anger management sessions, as arranged by the programme. When the department responds to SN's email, reviewing the coverage schedule and doing a root-cause analysis, it concludes that SN's claims are unfounded. Even if individual errors had occurred, there is no evidence of a systemic problem or of a general risk to the public.

For the next few months, SN exhibits appropriately professional behaviour and even nursing staff comment on his change in attitude. After the remediation period ends, SN moves on to his fourth year of training. As he assumes more responsibility, he seems to have limited patience for questions from junior residents and interns. One afternoon he tells the medical students on his team to leave early since they are 'useless', and the next day he criticises them for failing to complete their work. Later that week, the programme director is informed that, on two separate occasions, SN placed his hands on an intern's shoulders and moved her out of the way so that he could approach a patient's bedside. The programme director reinstitutes a 2-month remediation period, again focusing on professionalism, communication and respect for members of the team. SN seems contrite and his demeanour with junior residents and medical students seems to improve.

While on remediation, SN receives notice of an award to a prestigious fellowship programme at another institution. He receives uniformly glowing evaluations for most of this last year of training, and the senior medical staff consider him to be something of a rising star. One week short of completing his remediation period, however, SN gets into a violent disagreement with a nurse in the operating room. When the nurse points out that he is about to operate on the patient's wrong side, he grabs a surgical instrument and throws it at her, grazing her shoulder. He proceeds to shout insults and demands that she be removed. Unable to calm down, SN is the one who is escorted out, and that afternoon, over the protestations of a number of members of the department, SN is summarily suspended. Nonetheless, SN is allowed to return to work on probation for the final months in the programme, but he is warned that any single incidence of unprofessional behaviour will result in immediate dismissal.

SN appeals his suspension and probation. The Appeals Committee reviews his record and interviews witnesses to the recent incident, as well as supervisors and other individuals with information that is relevant to suspension and probation decisions. During his hearing, SN refers back to his complaints about inadequate coverage on the post-operative units and problems with nursing staff. He claims that his disciplinary action is retaliation for raising these issues about patient safety. The Appeals Committee considers his claims about coverage and nursing staff and reviews the department's response. The committee does not see SN as a legitimate whistle-blower, nor does it accept that the programme's actions were retaliatory.

A number of peers and supervising physicians testify at his hearing stressing SN's talent and intelligence. His supporters emphasise that having this indelible mark on his record would have negative repercussions for his career. The committee struggles with this aspect of the case, but the record cannot be erased, and the suspension and probation actions are upheld. While SN satisfactorily completes the programme with no further lapses in professionalism, the disciplinary actions of suspension and probation are duly reported to the state licensing authority. SN is required to notify the fellowship programme about the suspension and probation, and in future, he will be required to disclose this record of disciplinary action on all applications for state licensure and hospital staff privileges.

Questions

- How often is this type of behaviour tolerated in the operating room, and should SN's behaviour be excused on account of his reputation as an excellent surgeon?
- Was the programme director imposing remediation and formal discipline to address legitimate concerns, or were these actions a defence against future claims by house and/or nursing staff?

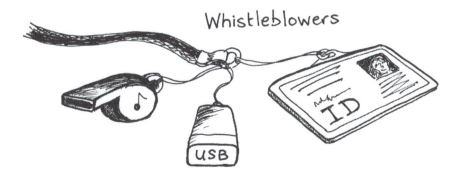

- How significant was SN's response to the death of a patient? Should this have triggered a more supportive response to help him learn how to handle difficult outcomes?
- What are the long-term repercussions of the final disciplinary action? Is this too severe?
- What additional actions would have been necessary for SN to be treated as a true and genuine whistle-blower?

Discussion

A talented professional may be given latitude in the area of interpersonal communication when 'people skills' seem secondary to brilliant diagnostic or surgical skills. Not only may a programme director face the challenge of training a young physician with deficits in professionalism due to personality, youth and inexperience but also there may be the obstacle of mentors or role models in the department, who themselves fail to uphold appropriate standards of professional behaviour. Furthermore, attempts to remediate a trainee's performance may be hindered by supervisors who do not acknowledge the problem. In this case, the programme director developed remediation plans and ultimately imposed disciplinary action, but the events precipitating those decisions were fairly dramatic and could have had serious consequences. The programme director had real concerns about future grievances from staff and patients related to SN's behaviour. The steps taken were motivated by the need to protect the well-being of patients and staff and the need to push SN to conform to the standards of professionalism for his own development as a physician.

The postgraduate curriculum, in contrast to medical school, does not formally provide an elective focused on opportunities to develop coping skills and accommodate grief related to poor patient outcomes and other emotional events linked to patient care. However, there is a designated psychiatrist available to all postgraduate trainees at no charge, to whom the residents and fellows can turn for support and treatment on a strictly confidential basis. The programme director probably should have referred SN for consultation with the psychiatrist on a voluntary basis when his reaction to stressful situations first gave rise to concern.

In order for SN to be a true whistle-blower, he would genuinely have to believe his stated concerns about post-operative coverage by medical staff and nursing incompetence, and these concerns would have to have merit as a risk to public health. In addition, his claim as a whistle-blower necessitates a link between the disciplinary action and his threat to report or publicise his allegations. Sufficient steps were taken to ensure that none of these conditions applied.

Summary

- SN was verbally abusive and physically inappropriate with co-residents and hospital staff. Remediation plans were ineffective in preventing the last breach of professionalism, and it was unclear whether suspension and probation would have a lasting impact on his behaviour. Dismissal could have been a more appropriate response.

- Corrective actions and disciplinary measures imposed were warranted by SN's unprofessional behaviour. Furthermore, he satisfied the terms of his probation plan and exhibited respect for staff until near the point of graduation. Concerns remained that SN could again 'snap' at some point in the future.

- SN's disrespect for trainees and nursing staff, and his repeated bouts of unchecked anger created an unsafe environment for staff and patients.

- The dramatic contrast between SN's clinical skills and interpersonal skills exemplifies a challenge to supervisors and programme directors. Training and education programmes have to address professional behaviours as well as clinical skills.

- Following the disciplinary protocol was crucial in this case.

- The state licensing board was notified and would be expected to investigate the events leading to disciplinary action.

- Guidelines did not play a part in this case.

CASE 10

An international medical graduate is showing poor reasoning and judgement.

Outline

TI is a resident in the paediatric residency training programme. He attended medical school in another country prior to coming to the United States and spending time working in a research lab at an academic medical centre. When he eventually secured a place in the training programme he went on to have a distinguished academic record, with accolades for his work in the lab and several published papers. Because of the years spent away from a clinical setting, his programme director expected a period of adjustment; however, by the end of TI's first year, his supervisors and peers report significant deficits in both clinical skill and professionalism, and on ward rounds he often has trouble presenting cases. TI seems overly focused on certain details, which are not necessarily pertinent to the case, and he tends to jump to conclusions about a diagnosis, without paying attention to potentially significant symptoms or test results.

Instead of accepting constructive criticism, he becomes defensive about his analysis and treatment recommendations. These concerns lead to a remediation period focusing on organisation and presentation skills. During this period, TI's presentations improve, but he continues to resist efforts from his supervisors to help him properly analyse the medical data before making decisions about treatment. A remediation period is put in place for 2 months, during which TI seems more open to feedback. His performance improves and he is then allowed to resume normal practice.

However, during the second year, TI's performance is uneven. He receives glowing evaluations from some supervisors and peers, but others report uncertainty about whether TI appropriately raises red flags when a patient's symptoms indicate a potentially serious condition. Again, members of staff are put off by his refusal to consider alternative viewpoints. When supervisors question his conclusions or thought process, he maintains an unshakable confidence regarding his perspective on the patient's illness and medical needs. Numerous members of the hospital's medical and nursing staff note his brusque and at times dismissive attitude. In spite of these concerns, TI is not placed on remediation again, because his programme director believes that clinically he is heading in the right direction. In addition, an article about the research project he was worked on is selected for publication in a prestigious journal.

There is speculation that his demeanour might be attributable to cultural differences rather than flaws in his professionalism. At the beginning of his third year, when the resident assumes responsibility for supervising interns and running the team, a chief resident contacts the programme director with a number of concerns. TI's admission notes are alarmingly brief, his interns complain that he does not conduct formal rounds or give them enough guidance and, on one occasion, TI did not respond to numerous pages from an intern having difficulty managing a very sick patient. A supervising faculty member notes that TI's case presentations in clinic are poor and he lacks interest in this 'less sick' group of outpatients. Additionally, there is at least one patient for whom TI fails to call a timely specialist consult, even though the patient suffers no medical deterioration due to the delay. Finally, after a night when TI was on call in the paediatric intensive care unit (PICU), his intern reports that without giving night-time instructions to the intern TI simply left the intern with his pager number and went to sleep.

The intern was extremely anxious that night and when initially unable to reach TI by pager, he contacted the fellow on call, who came into the hospital to assist with two very sick patients. Upon learning of this night in the PICU, the programme director suspends TI because she believes that he was compromising patient safety and welfare. During the suspension period, a handful of interns and junior residents who had worked with TI put their names on a group email to the programme director, claiming that on several occasions they have been embarrassed in front of others by TI's demeaning comments, and, individually, they have been subjected to his bouts of anger and insults. After reviewing this email and the supervisor evaluations for TI, many of which were quite positive, and investigating the events in the PICU, the programme director imposes a 3-month probation period, outlining goals and objectives focusing heavily on professionalism, clearly stating that non-promotion or dismissal is a likely result if TI does not satisfy the terms of probation.

TI appeals his suspension and probation. However, prior to the conclusion of his appeal and before the end of the probation period, TI resigns from the programme. In his resignation letter to the programme director, he outlines his numerous academic accomplishments and refutes the data presented in his evaluations and patient records with his own interpretation of the facts. He adamantly defends every clinical judgement that had been questioned or criticised by the programme. He denies any difficulty in relating to the interns and criticises them for being too sensitive to his constructive criticism and too timid by not asking for help.

In addition, TI accuses the programme director of violating anti-discrimination laws, based on his age and national origin. He makes allegations that the programme is biased against his national origin, and it unfairly held him to a higher standard in order to disparage the quality of medical training he had received in his home country. In spite of these claims, TI stops short of suing the institution. Because TI resigns in lieu of facing further disciplinary action, the institution is obliged to report this to state licensing authorities.

Questions

- Were concerns about TI's clinical judgement initially minimised due to his academic record and research achievements? Are academic pursuits and professional behaviour in clinical settings at odds?
- How significant was TI's perceived 'superior' attitude? Should this have triggered suspicion about TI's clinical competence?
- Could TI's more mature age have caused his supervisors and peers to be more or less deferential to his opinions than those of his peers?
- How significant was TI's unavailability to and seeming lack of interest in teaching his interns? How could this have affected patient care?
- Are interns and junior residents more or less likely to raise real concerns about senior residents? When such complaints are made, are they taken seriously or discounted?
- If TI had raised claims of unlawful discrimination at an internal appeal hearing, what type of inquiry into those claims would have been appropriate in determining whether to uphold or overturn the disciplinary actions?

Discussion

Assessing a resident who has an accomplished research career may present a challenge when programme directors either find themselves overly impressed by such achievements or feel pressure from influential faculty members who have an interest in the success of the resident. Additionally, a programme director may be hesitant in addressing areas in need of improvement in a more mature trainee with a different cultural background and foreign training. The goal of excellence in training and the primary concern of patient safety may seem so obvious that a talented trainee may too easily be forgiven for what is perceived as mere egoism.

In spite of these challenges, the programme director attempts to address TI's weaknesses with a remediation plan, and while TI was intellectually capable of improving, his inconsistent performance put the programme in a difficult situation. Ultimately, the risk to patient safety created by his lack of professionalism forced the programme to take a firm stand. Rather than serving as a wake-up call to TI, his suspension marked the end of his commitment to clinical training. TI had the opportunity on probation to prove his dedication, but having his competence openly questioned seemed to be too devastating a blow to his ego.

Although clinical concerns persisted, the most significant factor leading to TI's failure was linked to professionalism. The common thread throughout his evaluations was lack of recognition of his deficiencies and refusal to accept feedback. His defensive attitude and unwillingness to consider alternative viewpoints interfered with the possibility of meaningful improvement. As a senior resident, his attitude towards the junior members of the team and his unavailability, coupled with his overconfidence, created a liability to the programme as a whole. Upon TI's decision to resign, the suspension and probation actions were deemed final, with the resignation and disciplinary actions having to be reported to the state licensing authority.

Summary

- The most significant problem arising in this case was TI's unwillingness to take feedback from his supervisors and his inability to accept that, in spite of demonstrated intelligence and academic achievements, he needed to improve his clinical skills and professional behaviour.
- We believe that the disciplinary actions taken were fair, and that in the light of TI's poor interpersonal skills and lack of insight into the level of professionalism required to function in a clinical setting, his decision to terminate clinical training was probably best for both him and the programme.
- While no patients were harmed, the programme director correctly viewed TI's behaviour as posing a risk to patient safety. Jumping to

clinical conclusions and refusing to consider opinions of peers and supervisors could have had serious consequences, as could inadequately supervising interns, creating a barrier to communication and displaying a demeaning and insulting attitude.

- This case provides a warning against giving too much weight to academic accomplishments preceding entrance into a clinical training programme. Supervisors and programme directors must remain focused on clinical skill and professional behaviour appropriate to the patient care setting. If problems arise, all members of the team, including interns and medical students, should be given an opportunity to be heard.

- Following disciplinary protocol was critical in ferreting out this resident's weaknesses. Unfortunately, rather than serving as an appropriate corrective action, as more focus was placed on his lapses in professionalism, his resistance to improvement increased.

- If TI stayed in the United States, the state licensing board would be expected to investigate the circumstances surrounding his resignation from training by requesting a copy of his personnel file and potentially interviewing witnesses.

- No particular local or national guidelines were used in addressing concerns raised by TI's behaviour.

CASE 11

A junior doctor, accused of being dishonest, threatens to 'expose' a senior colleague.

Outline

PM is an intern (first-year resident) in the internal medicine residency training programme. During her first few months in the programme, her programme director receives a few reports of concern about PM's professionalism. Specifically, PM's co-residents complain that they suspected that at times she had not been truthful about certain tasks having been completed, such as diagnostic tests ordered or patients examined. There are no reports of patient harm or evidence of outright lying. Nonetheless, the programme director meets with PM to raise these issues and counsel her regarding professionalism.

The programme director makes it clear that there is an absolute expectation of truthfulness of every member of the medical team, even at the risk of admitting delays or errors. PM denies any dishonesty and claims that her peers are mistaken and perhaps unfairly judging her because they resent having recently been asked to cover her on-call schedule due to her brief absence relating to a death in her family. The programme director assures her that he would remain alert to any confounding interpersonal issues among the house staff, stating that PM needs to take these concerns seriously and that further lapses in professionalism would not be tolerated.

At the end of the first 3 months of training, upon receiving the first set of written evaluations from PM's supervisors and peers, the programme director discovers that concerns about PM's truthfulness persist among members of the house staff and medical staff, as well as nursing staff. Again, there are no reports of patient harm, but more than one resident provides an example of doing a ward round with PM and discovering her complete lack of familiarity with clinical facts about a patient for whom she had written a note and insisted she had examined that morning.

The programme director follows up with a few faculty members who had supervised PM and consults with the house staff office. The programme director believes that, because of the inconclusive nature of the scenarios reported and the strong praise PM received from a trusted faculty member, a formal remediation plan rather than a summary suspension would be most appropriate. The programme director is also aware that PM had witnessed him out on a date one evening with another female resident (trainee), and he wants to keep this private.

The programme director meets with PM and provides her with a written warning and plan of remediation. The plan sets forth the expectations of the programme in terms of professionalism and goals to be met, including satisfactory ratings on all written peer and supervisor evaluations and no reports of concern about PM's professionalism from any source at the hospital. PM continues to deny any wrongdoing, insisting that complaints are due to misunderstandings and personal gripes among her peers. She threatens to expose the programme director's secret relationship and refuses to sign an acknowledgement of the remediation plan, which she understands will be in effect for the next 3 months.

Five weeks into the remediation period, the programme director receives a distressing report that, the night before, during PM's rotation in the emergency department, PM brought a friend dressed in scrubs to observe her while she cared for patients. A co-intern had alerted the chief resident that PM had mentioned that her roommate had been in the emergency room (ER) overnight and assisted PM in caring for an injured patient. The programme director meets with PM and summarily suspends her, pending an investigation into the reported incident and a review of PM's performance during the start of her remediation period. At the programme director's request, PM provides a written response to the allegations about that night in the ER.

In her response, PM states that she believed that her roommate, Ms A, who was a volunteer at the hospital and who was considering a career in medicine, was permitted to shadow her in the ER, provided that she identified herself as a volunteer and received permission from the patients. PM claims that she introduced Ms A to the ER staff as a hospital volunteer and that no one questioned whether she was authorised to be there. PM denies that Ms A had assisted in bandaging or providing any direct patient care. PM accuses her co-intern of fabricating that aspect of his account so as to get PM into trouble. PM also claims that with the remediation plan and resulting rumours about her credibility, the programme is putting a 'target' on her back and that people are just waiting for her to fail. In her written statement PM expresses no remorse regarding the decision to bring her roommate into the ER that night and no recognition of her responsibility for her difficulties as a trainee.

In addition to reviewing PM's submission, the programme director questions eyewitnesses to verify that Ms A had been in the ER that night with PM. He also contacts the hospital's volunteer office and confirms that Ms A had applied to become a volunteer, but not until the day following PM's suspension. The programme director also examines the chart of the patient, who was allegedly bandaged with Ms A's assistance, and there is no record of consent for observation or indication of the observer's presence in PM's note. After consultation with the house staff office and upon recommendation by the programme director, the department chair dismisses PM from the training programme. PM appeals her suspension and dismissal to an internal hearing committee. During her hearing, PM claims that the programme director has been out to get her because she had threatened to expose a personal relationship with another resident in the programme. She insists that this person's motivation, credibility and professionalism ought to be questioned. Although she continues to deny any wrongdoing, the department's decision to dismiss PM from the programme is eventually upheld.

Questions

- Are concerns about truthfulness sufficient cause to place a resident on remediation or summary suspension? What types of untruths, if any, are more or less acceptable?
- Was the incident involving PM's roommate sufficient cause to suspend and then dismiss her from the training programme? What effect should the fabrication about Ms A's volunteer status have had on the choice of disciplinary action?
- In what way could the programme director's personal relationship with PM's co-resident have affected his judgement?
- Should the committee considering PM's appeal have considered her allegations about the programme director's relationship with the other resident when reviewing the disciplinary action?

- What standard of review would be appropriate to determine whether to overturn or uphold PM's dismissal?

Discussion

The difficulty in assessing interns often lies in the tendency of programme directors and supervising physicians to give a new trainee the benefit of the doubt even when problems become apparent. Residency training programmes draw from vastly different medical schools, as well as international programmes, and these discrepancies often rightly account for a programme's tolerance of a range of knowledge base, skill and other professional behaviours among trainees during the period of adjustment. Thereafter, a programme director may be confronted with a serious situation when a more complete picture of the 'weak' intern reveals either deficits in competencies or a pattern of behaviour that may ultimately put patients at risk and be difficult to correct.

In this case, the programme director appropriately imposed a remediation plan when concerns about the intern's professionalism arose. At this point it appeared that PM posed no risk to patient safety, and the accusations against her were somewhat inconclusive. However, PM's response to the warning and remediation (i.e. outright denial of any responsibility for possible misunderstandings, a refusal to sign the acknowledgement that she had received and understood as regards the written warning, and, finally, her threat to expose the programme director's personal relationship) should have given the programme director a strong suspicion that the remediation plan would not prove successful. The programme director had no choice but to suspend and ultimately dismiss PM, when her lapse in professional judgement caused her to invite her roommate into a patient care setting and then lie about the situation when she was caught.

PM's decision to appeal her suspension and dismissal to an internal committee, in accordance with due process, was understandable given the fact that without such a hearing, the dismissal would have been final and would have required a mandatory report being sent to the state licensing authority. This was the end result after the committee rendered its decision. While PM wanted to pursue a lawsuit against the institution and the programme director for wrongful termination, it would be unlikely that an experienced attorney would take on her case. Without evidence of retaliation against protected behaviour (e.g. whistle-blowing) or a compelling argument that the programme's action was arbitrary or in violation of an anti-discrimination statute, the courts generally give deference to academic training programmes when making decisions about disciplinary action.

Summary

- The most significant problem arising in this case was the lack of integrity exemplified by PM's persistent lying about matters ranging from the completion of minor duties to a serious violation of hospital policy and professional ethics.
- We believe that the outcome was fair and appropriate due to the seriousness of PM's transgressions.
- While no patient was harmed, the programme director, department chair and appeal committee were firm in the conviction that PM could not be trusted to care for patients and relay critical information to the medical team. She demonstrated repeated untruthfulness and lack of insight into the professionalism implications of her conduct.
- This case highlights the need for educators to be alert to complaints and poor evaluations about a trainee's behaviour, and the importance of following up on any identified concerns.[9]
- Disciplinary protocol must be followed when instituting a remediation plan or procedures for suspension and dismissal, otherwise the programme director could have denied her due process, and PM would have had grounds for challenging the disciplinary action.
- The state licensing board would be expected to investigate the circumstances surrounding PM's termination from training and the concerns about her professionalism when reviewing any future application for a medical licence.
- According to state law, the legal definition of professional misconduct underlies the significance of disciplinary action taken in this case, including PM's violation of confidentiality laws and a pattern of lying, which meet the definition of 'moral unfitness to practise medicine'.

CASE 12

A trainee who tries to cover up his mistakes claims he is a whistle-blower. *

Outline

LT, a second-year Foundation doctor, is working in the emergency department. His primary training was in Egypt, and in some respects he finds it difficult to adapt to the culture of the National Health Service; by his own admission, his spoken English is better than his written English. He has never had any *serious* problems, but, like many doctors, he does not like filing paperwork and he was

---

* While this is a fictionalised case, like others in this book, elements of the account are based on actual cases that are in the public domain.

recently criticised by Dr F, a senior house officer, for inaccurate and incomplete recording in the patient notes.

One morning LT arrives 30 minutes late for his shift, causing the house officer on the previous shift to have to stay late. He senses bad feelings and apologises, but then he acts as though distracted in some way. He enters in the notes of the first patient, Patient A, that a urinalysis had been performed (after being brought in with acute pain, and in a generally confused state); while bacterial cultures are running, LT prescribes broad-spectrum intravenous antibiotics. Dr F decides to transfer Patient A to the clinical assessment unit pending results of his tests. However, Dr F finds that, contrary to LT's notes, no urine sample appears to have been taken or sent to microbiology. Patient A, who is elderly with mild dementia, is unable to recall what did or did not happen. The delay may not harm the patient, but samples need to be taken and sent off and the discrepancy must be sorted.

The next day, Dr F tells his registrar about this incident and she in turn speaks to LT. He says it was a mistake and that he must have simply muddled up two patients' notes, but later that same day there is another incident in which his notes are not accurately recorded. In the second incident, Patient B comes to the emergency department with a friend, who claims that Patient B is severely depressed and needs urgent treatment. Patient B is happy to talk about his problems with LT, who does an initial assessment before ordering further investigations. However, LT wrongly records the name of the drug that Patient B had previously been given by his general practitioner. This error only comes to light several days later, by which time initial inquiries into the first incident imply that LT lied in order to cover up his mistake.

With two incidents occurring on the same day, the case escalates and hospital management temporarily suspend LT while an internal investigation is carried out. On further questioning, LT gives a less than accurate account of events that are later disproved. He claims he was just having a bad day and that nobody was harmed. He had had a row with his wife the night before and had spent the night on a friend's sofa. In LT's opinion, this was sufficient mitigation, and he promises that nothing like this will ever happen again.

Hospital governance then files a report saying that LT is dishonest and unreliable, and on public interest grounds they pass the report on to the General Medical Council (GMC). Because of concerns about probity as well as clinical competence, LT's case is eventually referred to a full hearing before a panel at the GMC. He still does not give an accurate record of what happened that day, but when confronted with written evidence from nursing staff and others, he finally owns up to having lied in order get himself out of trouble.

His behaviour is found to be incompatible with the standard expected of a doctor registered with the GMC, and he is found guilty of professional misconduct.

He is suspended for 9 months and prevented from working as a doctor during that time. He is advised to do further training in order to try to raise his standards and level of understanding; he complies with this recommendation, but during the period of suspension he travels to another deanery area to perform locum work with an agency that never bothers to check his registration.

He applies to the GMC to be reinstated on the register near the end of the period of suspension. By this time, LT is angry at the way this case has had such dire consequences in terms of his career; he claims that when first reported to the GMC, he had been victimised and bullied by management. In his view, they were trying to cover up for inadequacies in the way that the department was being run. He believes that the standard of care he provides is neither better nor worse than that of any of his peers; he says nothing about the 'moonlighting'. During his suspension he continued to have a training number with the deanery, meaning that his post could not be taken by anyone else, and that the hospital is left understaffed. By the time of the GMC panel decision, news of the case finds its way into the local media.

LT complied with the recommendations of the panel and undertook additional training, which he paid for out of the money that he earned as a locum. Nonetheless, he tries to make a serious point about the way the hospital is being run, which he thinks is putting the public at risk. He goes on to give an interview with a local newspaper to reinforce his point; this finds its way onto the front page and then into the hands of the GMC. At this point, LT's locum work comes to light, because someone reading the newspaper recognises the doctor's name; at the second GMC hearing, where he applies to be reinstated, LT is asked to explain his actions.

LT sees no connection between the fitness to practise inquiries and his right to voice concerns about a public service, and he has heard of other doctors working while suspended. Furthermore, he feels his actions are providing a public service by highlighting potentially dangerous practices, and that he should be regarded as a whistle-blower. He admits to his mistakes but says they were only minor, and he still thinks he has been harshly treated. The second GMC panel takes a dim view of LT's public utterances and feels that they show lack of judgement on his part, as well as a lack of insight. Furthermore, because of working while suspended by the regulator, the GMC panel determines that his name should be permanently erased from the register. LT then takes legal advice about applying to the High Court to lodge an appeal to try to have the decision overturned.

Questions

- How relevant is the reported domestic dispute in terms of it affecting his judgement and clinical performance?

- Has this doctor been the victim of workplace bullying?
- Has he really acted as a 'whistle-blower', and to what extent should his comments be taken seriously?
- Was the final decision too harsh?

Discussion

This case began with incidents that were fairly minor, and initially one sees no reason why this doctor's behaviour should ever need to be brought to the attention of the regulator. Most doctors who are facing internal disciplinary hearings would hopefully learn the lesson and make greater efforts (e.g. as regards note-taking); however, LT tried to cover his tracks and in so doing made the situation many times worse. The clinical lapse in his behaviour was easy to remediate; however, the probity aspect was more challenging, reflecting an underlying attitude that might be hard to address; persistent dishonesty reflects personality traits that may not be remediable. Furthermore, the greater the difficulty this doctor found himself in the harder he made things for himself, eventually trying to defend the indefensible. Working while suspended was the deal-breaker in terms of LT's future career as a doctor, and by the time of the second hearing, there was probably no other decision that the panel could have reached. Appealing the decision in court might be a case of throwing good money after bad, with very little chance of success.

Nonetheless, some doubts remain about how the hospital is being run, and junior doctors, who are on the front line, sometimes know more than their managers about day-to-day events in the department. Given that LT was bringing patient safety issues to public attention, it is hard to ignore these complaints, but had he acted more wisely and brought these issues to the attention of relevant authorities prior to having his own reputation being placed in jeopardy, he could, indeed, have been doing a public service.

Summary

- Probity and professionalism are the overarching issues in this case; questions of clinical competence were entirely secondary, even though they acted as an initial trigger for the local investigation.
- We think the final outcome was fair and proportionate, brought upon by LT's own behaviour. Everything relating to the initial complaint would have gone away had LT acted professionally and showed insight (instead of a tendency to deceive).
- Patient safety was important with respect to the poor note-taking; public protection was also important, even though no direct harm was caused to patients. LT had ample opportunity to put things right early and

come clean; failure to do so and working while under suspension were inexcusable, even though locum fees were used to fund further training.

- International medical graduates who land in difficulties with the regulator may do so because of differences in professional culture and training. While this does not excuse LT's behaviour, from an educational perspective it is something that supervisors need to bear in mind.
- Protocol was not really an issue in this case.
- Most complaints against doctors are dealt with at the local level, and the senior house office in this case was right to bring things to the attention of his registrar; in turn, had she not brought things to the attention of human resources, she herself might have been negligent for failing to act appropriately in protecting patient safety.
- In the United Kingdom the duties of a doctor are well known, and doctors are beholden to know about and adhere as best they can to core guidance issued by the GMC.[10]

CASE 13

A medical student has a pattern of non-attendance and dishonesty.

Outline

A final-year medical student, known to everyone as AY, has a reputation with the tutors as being very personable; however, he does not always do well in his exams and he often asks for extra time with handing in assignments. This recurring pattern comes to a head when he fails to turn up for a written exam without letting anyone know where he is. When challenged by an associate dean at the medical school he says that he had been unwell that day and had sent a message in through a friend. When asked for corroboration, he gives the name of a fellow medical student, ML, who is his girlfriend; when questioned on her own, ML admits that she had been asked to cover for AY, but she didn't want to land herself in trouble, which is why she did not follow through with AY's request.

A disciplinary committee for AY is convened and a hearing date set. By this point, AY has found out that ML had provided evidence to the effect that he was being dishonest, which results in their break-up. AY does not show up for the hearing, and in absentia he is temporarily excluded from the school for unprofessional conduct; as a consequence, he will be prevented from completing his degree on time.[*]

---

[*] NB: The dean is the person responsible for writing a reference in support of this candidate and all residency applications; therefore, not only would AY *not* graduate on time but also when (and if) he did complete his degree, he would be reliant on a good reference for getting accepted on to an intern programme.

AY's father is a lawyer, and a partner from his firm writes to the school, challenging his suspension. Mr P, the attorney, claims that AY has been the victim of unfair discrimination, because the student suffered from attention deficit hyperactivity disorder (ADHD), making it difficult for him to meet deadlines and work well under pressure. Mr P claims that ML was the one who was lying and that she had simply forgotten to say anything to anyone about the exam, resulting in the 'unexplained absence' being recorded for AY.

The school replies, saying that they have no record of AY having ADHD, and if this is new evidence, it should have been submitted at the right time through the proper channels. AY's conduct, in the school's view, was unprofessional and could bring the profession into disrepute. Predictably, AY is unhappy with the decision and decides to lodge an appeal. Mr P argues that the medical school has failed to respect AY's human rights and, what is more, if the decision is not overturned on appeal, they will file a lawsuit seeking monetary compensation for the delay to the start of his career, reimbursement of legal costs and an undertaking that the university provide a favourable reference.

Mr P points out that 6 weeks previously, AY's maternal grandmother, a Palestinian woman living in the West Bank, had been injured in a bombing raid. On the day of the exam, AY had a call from his mother saying that his grandmother was not expected to recover. This was the real reason for his absence, and, while avoiding the accusation of racism, there is an implication in the letter that the school was acting in a prejudicial way towards this student because of his family's ethnicity.

An appeal hearing is duly scheduled in line with university procedures. This time AY does appear, along with his attorney; however, the decision does not go in their favour. The appeal is rejected and the school's position is upheld. He is not reinstated or given an immediate chance to retake the exam, and as a result of the temporary suspension he will be unable to graduate on time. The dean takes the view that this is the only sensible outcome, and the school argues that public interest has to be respected and that there are important professional implications arising from this case. The new evidence is not valid, as it was not introduced at the appropriate time or in the appointed way; AY had ample opportunity to defend his case and explain any mitigating circumstances.

Two days later the dean receives a letter stating that Mr P was applying to the court to try to have the judgement overturned. They do not accept that AY had not acted in an inappropriate or unprofessional way; he had simply been under pressure and, in addition, he has a recognised learning disability that has not been taken into account. This case causes nervousness among senior members of staff, some of whom advocate that for the sake of damage limitation, the case should be settled out of court. However, the dean and the school's lawyers think otherwise, and their view prevails.

At the hearing before a circuit court judge, the full circumstances surrounding this case are heard. When summing up, the judge says that Mr P's arguments are not relevant, as the school had followed its own legally correct procedures; as a result, the medical school's position is again upheld. By this time, the school has been put through a great deal of expense and trouble; the judge decides that each party should pay its own costs.

Questions

- To what extent do you think this case is about human rights?
- What steps (if any) could the school take to try to prevent a similar case from arising in the future?
- Disability plays a part in this case; to what extent does a diagnosis of ADHD change how professionalism should be judged and enforced?
- How relevant is the implication of racial prejudice in Mr P's letter to the school?

Discussion

This case has many layers. Central to the case was AY's unprofessional behaviour. Everything else was secondary, and because the school acted properly and adhered to its own practices and procedures, ultimately there was little that AY or his family lawyer could do. The challenge to the school for failing to respect AY's human rights was probably opportunistic; if the student had had a genuine disability then proper channels would have been followed, and the school would almost certainly have taken this into account during exams. However, these claims were found to be without foundation.

The ethnic aspect of the case, while in some respects real, was not relevant and it merely had the effect of making the case more difficult for members of faculty, and possibly even for the court. If AY had received bad news on the day of the exam, he should have rung in and asked to be allowed to take the exam another day. This initial indiscretion was compounded by his failure to appear at the first hearing, as well as asking his girlfriend to lie on his behalf. Probity was the real issue, not human rights. Cases that give rise to allegations involving human rights, and particularly cases that include mention of race, almost by definition become high stakes for everyone involved. A school may be tempted to cave in and reach a settlement prior to going to court on grounds of expediency. It requires strong nerves on the part of key members of faculty to stand their ground.*

---

* A ruling in the case of Halpern versus Wake Forest University Health Sciences, 2010, US District Lexis 77771, argues that the court has a duty to strike a balance 'between the statutory rights of the handicapped to be integrated into society and the legitimate interests of federal grantees in preserving the integrity of their program' (§29).

Most medical school cohorts have students coming from many different ethnic backgrounds, and quite possibly one or two students have family members living in politically difficult regions of the world. Once again, if this were indeed a matter of genuine concern it should and could have been addressed at an earlier time (e.g. via student support). Had ML acted differently, the case could have been rather more difficult in terms of deciding who was telling the truth. If she had lied to protect her boyfriend, there would have also been consequences for her career, had this come to light.

Summary

- This student acted in a way that would have been wholly unacceptable from a qualified, practising clinician. AY may have created a good impression with his tutors, but when under pressure he proved unreliable and dishonest.
- While attempts were made to prove unfairness, with unspoken allegations of racial prejudice and disability, nothing was substantiated and the final outcome was in all probability correct.
- Questions of patient safety and public protection were more implied than explicit in terms of this student's behaviour. However, when a medical student displays behavioural characteristics such as these and they go unchecked, it has potentially damaging consequences, including showing other students that they can 'get away' with all kinds of behaviour.
- Staff development is always important, and if a school does not have enough suitably trained people able to respond carefully and critically in situations such as this, it could be difficult for a school to achieve a satisfactory outcome.
- There is very little that a school can do to prevent such cases from happening except to make sure practices and procedures are robust, clearly stated, and carefully followed.
- Quality assurance teams should make sure that a school has appropriate policies and procedures in place. Reacting to a situation after a difficulty has arisen is much more difficult for all concerned, and could potentially result in this student winning on appeal or in court.
- In this case, there were no issues directly relating to guidelines.

CASE 14

A junior doctor, with a history of poor performance, starts failing assessments.

Outline

A 24-year-old Foundation year 1 doctor, TP, is reported by his first rotation supervisor to have odd interpersonal skills and to be behaving 'strangely' at work. His attendance is reasonable, but he is often sloppily dressed and unkempt, and his work 'efficiency' is below normal because of poor organisational skills. He has a tendency to be rather obsessive with certain tasks while apparently ignoring or forgetting others, and he is so slow that he often does not complete his duties within normal shift hours. His communication style with patients is blunt, and other trainees have to check his work and fill in gaps or repeat poorly executed tasks (even though he often stays late with the aim of trying to complete these tasks).

His knowledge and skills appear reasonable, but it soon becomes obvious that he will fail his in-training assessment (ITA). The situation angers the supervising consultant because TP was a medical student at that hospital and was well known as a poor performer, and yet the medical school 'allowed him to graduate'. The consultant questions why they did not do their job properly, and when he tries to discuss the issues with TP, he feels that he is getting nowhere. While TP is pleasant, open about his weaknesses and willing to try to improve, he does not seem *able* to improve. TP is referred to the Foundation Programme Committee, which includes senior representation from the medical school. He is therefore well known to several members of the committee, who had been anxious about him during medical school, particularly during the clinical years. However, he always managed to pass clinical assessments and there was no mechanism available for preventing his progress.

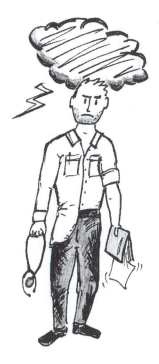

He is provided with additional support, including guidance on how to organise himself, but all that seems to achieve is to 'help him over the line' rather than lead to any improvement in skills. TP is eventually required to have health checks, including a psychiatric assessment, which indicates that he has a mild degree of autism. He continues in the Foundation Programme but he fails all of his in-training assessments and has to repeat the year.

Questions

- How has this situation arisen? Was the medical school wrong to allow him to graduate?
- Is this primarily a problem of health or of conduct? If the former, does this count as a disability; if the latter, what action is appropriate?
- Should TP have done his Foundation training at a different hospital so that his reputation did not precede him?
- Is it fair to make him repeat the year if the behaviours are not remediable?

Discussion

This case provides an example of a weakness that becomes especially pronounced when the individual concerned has to function independently (i.e. in the workplace). Getting by as a student is not the same as getting by in the workplace, and while the medical school no doubt followed procedure in allowing TP to graduate, this did not adequately prepare him for work. This case is not about apportioning blame; rather, it is about finding ways to try to prevent students with difficulties such as these from failing, especially in the workplace. Had he been diagnosed with autism *earlier* in his undergraduate career, it might have led to more appropriate support. This case possibly lies at the borderline of legality because the root cause of the problem was a health issue over which TP had no control, and clearly it would be unlawful for an employer to discriminate unreasonably on grounds of disability. Furthermore, as a syndrome covering a spectrum of problems, autism can be difficult to detect and treat. Employers can do their best to provide necessary support, but ultimately TP has to be capable of performing to an acceptable standard if he is to complete his basic training.

A first-year Foundation doctor is expected to have an opportunity to sort problems and make necessary transitions. This is built into the system, in that newly qualified doctors in the United Kingdom do not have *full* registration at the General Medical Council. In addition to the training provider, the medical school from which a student graduates retains the responsibility for signing off on doctors who satisfactorily complete the first year of training. A final-year undergraduate may be immersed in the workplace environment but this does not necessarily make the transition easier, and in cases where this process does not work effectively, it potentially calls into question the reliability of workplace-based assessments.

One of the strengths of the Foundation school model is joint medical school and National Health Service responsibility for trainees, and information can readily be shared between the university and the National Health Service employer. The formal mechanism is a 'transfer of information' form, which must be completed by each graduate and signed off by the medical school, a process that generally avoids concerns over confidentiality. Furthermore, if a doctor remains in the same geographical area, it is possible that some of the same people will be responsible for supervision and assessment across the transition from student to junior doctor.

The problem in this case is mainly one of health, but it is a problem that has a profound effect on professionalism. While it may not be possible to remedy the underlying health issue, it is imperative for each graduate to be able to meet the expected standard in terms of professionalism. Having an ineffective member of a team who cannot be left to work independently is damaging to everyone, and the doctor in question is unlikely to earn trust from his colleagues, to say nothing about the communication difficulties that he experiences with his patients.

Questions of patient safety are never far away, and there could well be risks to patients if TP continues to underperform. If he did eventually complete his Foundation training, an additional question arises as to how likely it is that he will get accepted on to a postgraduate specialty programme. This could be potentially difficult for this person, since his weaknesses are likely to impair his performance across *all* specialties. Aside from the issue of protecting patients, ultimately nobody wants a junior doctor to be set up to fail, and if one lacks the skills needed in order to be a successful practising clinician, an alternative career that utilises a degree in medicine should perhaps be considered.

Summary

- This case highlights the difficulty in separating out issues of professionalism from personal health. The professionalism aspect was fundamental but should not be viewed in isolation.
- Repeating the year was probably the only outcome, especially in that the underlying problem had not come to light earlier; however, this solution would not be fair to TP if all it does is postpone matters, leaving them for another committee to have to address later.
- The case of TP poses no problems in terms of public protection; however, patient safety could well be an issue when, or if, he reaches the stage of working more independently.
- If personality problems show up in medical school, supporting a

student to a minimum level whereby he or she passes exams may be an inadequate response without first considering what is behind the behaviour and implications for the student's future training and career.

- Good communication between the medical school and Foundation Programme is crucial; this ought to limit uncertainty about how information is shared.
- Problems highlighted in this case do not concern the regulator and can be dealt with effectively at local level.
- Guidelines were not an issue in this case.

CASE 15

A medical student is caught on camera stealing equipment from the hospital.

Outline

CA, a third-year medical student, is caught on hospital security cameras removing a portable ultrasound machine from a room, taking it down a long series of corridors, leaving by an unguarded back exit of the hospital and loading it into a car. The theft is confirmed the next morning, and security tapes clearly show the student's car licence plate. Because the suspect is a medical student, the dean of students is called and told about the situation. The dean makes an urgent appointment to see the student and when the issue of the theft is raised, CA quickly becomes anxious and red-faced and he starts sweating profusely while absolutely denying having anything to do with the theft. The dean of students then asks the hospital chief of security to produce the videotape on which CA's face is clearly visible. Confronted with the evidence CA breaks down in tears and admits the theft.

He goes on to describe his motivation, which stems from concern that his pregnant wife may be carrying a baby with a birth defect. This concern had been bothering him since an obstetrics–gynaecology rotation when he saw two women delivering babies with congenital defects. Having recently completed a tutorial on ultrasound, he planned to do weekly ultrasound scans so as to make sure that his wife's foetus is normal. 'I'm not a thief', he repeats over and over during the interview, and he again breaks down in tears. He goes on to explain that once his child was born he planned to return the ultrasound machine to the hospital. When asked, 'why not ask your wife's obstetrician to perform the scans?' he says that the obstetrician thought that frequent tests were not indicated in his wife's case, since the result of the ultrasound that was performed on his wife during a prenatal visit was entirely normal.

The dean of students reviews the student's progress through medical school. He was admitted after graduating from college at the top of his class, earning very high grades on the standardised premedical (Medical College Admissions Test) examination. CA did well in preclinical training and his performance on his clinical rotations was notable for his having received honours-level evaluations on most rotations. Although he is described as being somewhat reserved, he is also described as a team player, and no concerns about his professional behaviour were raised prior to this event. After conferring with legal counsel, the dean of students places CA on 'administrative leave' pending a formal hearing by the Medical Student Progress Committee (MSPC). The hospital expresses the view that it does not wish to press criminal charges, preferring instead to leave formal investigation and disciplinary proceedings up to the medical school.

The MSPC is made up of faculty members who meet regularly to discuss student issues; medical students are not represented, and the committee ultimately reports to the dean. The committee chairperson gives an account of the incident, and while the committee members consider theft of medical equipment to be 'seriously unprofessional conduct', the discussion quickly turns to whether or not CA has a mental health disorder; in their view this could be the cause of his preoccupation with his wife's pregnancy and his unwillingness to accept the reassurances from her doctor. The MSPC recommends a psychiatric evaluation at the university health centre before making any further judgement. At the next meeting of the committee, it is revealed that CA did not follow up and make an appointment, and hence there is no psychiatric report. The dean of students straight away calls CA in for a meeting; CA says, 'I'm not ill and I really don't want to have to go for psychiatric evaluation'. However, CA is told politely but firmly that he will have to comply, and that until he agrees he will remain on administrative leave. Several days after this meeting, the dean of students receives a call from a lawyer stating that she has been retained by the student and is asking for copies of CA's academic record.

The MSPC asks for a report from the student's advisor, who contacts CA by phone. The relationship he has with his advisor is generally good, but during the call CA sounds depressed and breaks down in tears, saying that this incident has seriously affected his sleep, appetite and concentration. CA reluctantly accepts that there is a problem; he agrees to have a psychiatric evaluation and makes an appointment to be seen at the health centre. CA is diagnosed as having depression with psychotic features and he is started on medication and supportive psychotherapy. However, his condition continues to deteriorate, and after consistently talking about killing himself as a way of being punished for his behaviour, he is briefly hospitalised. CA responds well to treatment, his baby is born healthy, and 8 months later he reports that he is interested in resuming his education. His treating psychiatrist provides a letter that is fully supportive of his resuming training, and nothing further is heard from CA's lawyer.

The MSPC meets again and feels that CA's unprofessional behaviour needs to be understood in the context of his mental illness, and that since his medical condition is now stable he should be allowed to return to medical school. No specific remediation plan regarding his unprofessional behaviour is in place, although the committee asks the dean of students and CA's advisor to talk with the student about the importance of continuing psychiatric treatment and learning how to manage professional responsibilities in the context of having a mental disorder.

The student does well in his remaining rotations and eventually graduates from medical school. During the process of applying for residency training, CA voluntarily discloses in his personal statement that he has a mood disorder, noting that he has been in treatment, and that he has been successful in managing the situation. Because it relates to an illness, his unprofessional conduct is not openly acknowledged in the letter that documents the student's progress through medical school and accompanies his residency applications (called the *Medical Student Performance Evaluation* [MSPE] or the *Dean's Letter*). When asked in his application to explain an interruption in his education he notes that his leave of absence was on medical grounds. Because in many respects he is otherwise a good student with many strong attributes, CA eventually matches at a prestigious residency programme. Follow-up suggests that he continues to do well, without any evidence of further unprofessional conduct.

Questions

- Is it reasonable for a school to insist that a student such as CA is referred for psychiatric evaluation?
- How much tolerance should a school show towards someone with a mental health impairment, especially when an unlawful act has been committed?
- Is it right that the student record in this case refers to a medical problem but not to unprofessional (or potentially criminal) behaviour?
- To what extent can CA's privacy of medical information be protected during this process?
- Is disability an issue in this case, and should professionalism be judged according to differing standards as against someone without a mental health impairment?

Discussion

Education leaders and academic committees charged with adjudicating issues of professionalism are often faced with the issue of whether a trainee has a mental health disorder that might explain his or her unprofessional conduct. In this instance, the Medical School Progress Committee (a version of which is required by the Licensing Committee for Medical Education, which regulates medical education in the United States) feels that there is good evidence suggesting that the student's unprofessional behaviour is due to him having a mental illness. However, this is not without controversy, because there will be nothing in the record to show that CA faced a disciplinary hearing and had a period of suspension following the matter of the theft.

While extended leave turned into medical leave, it did not start out that way, and had CA encountered further problems during his residency training, the prior information would have been crucial evidence in terms of establishing traits of behaviour. The end result turned out well and was in the student's favour; while nobody was actually put at risk, the case illustrates well the principle of overlapping areas of concern, and how it is often difficult to identify and separate health issues from underlying problems of behaviour. Had hospital administrators taken a different line and pressed for charges, depending on the adjudication of those charges, CA may have been unable to complete his medical education, with events taking a very different path.

Because of the high frequency in which mental illness plays a role in unprofessional behaviour, a progress committee may want to ensure that they have at least one member who is a psychiatrist. The dean of students could do well to maintain a close working relationship with the mental health division at the university health service; this should not be problematic, since the relationship with the mental health division explicitly excludes any details of student treatments, and so confidentiality in the therapeutic relationship ought to be preserved.

If a 'fitness to serve' evaluation is needed (or 'fitness to practise'), a psychiatrist *not* involved with the student's care would be called upon for an opinion. Local procedures must aim to eliminate potential conflicts of interest and to strive to preserve confidentiality in the therapeutic relationship. Either a fitness to serve evaluation would include a recommendation from a student's treating physician or the evaluation would come from the director of mental health services at the health plan. In that case, if the treatment is successful and the student is able to return to full function without significant residual symptoms, then the outcome can be considered good. However, full recovery is not always achievable, and trainees may continue to demonstrate significant symptoms of mental illness, which can compromise their ability to fully manage their professional duties. For example, depression may cause slowed thinking or concentration problems, or a manic episode may come on suddenly and cause a student to become agitated and grandiose about their medical knowledge or abilities. Both these situations could imperil patient care.

Managing situations in which mental illness continues to impair professional behaviour is inherently complicated. In the United States, trainees may declare that they have a disability, which under disability law mandates the provision of suitable 'accommodations'. This is a formal process, managed by a special office at the university, and if a student declares a disability that has been documented by a licensed medical provider, then education leaders must attempt to provide 'reasonable accommodations' for the student in order to give him or her the best possible chance to manage the illness and continue with professional training. 'Reasonable accommodations' are defined by a professional school's technical standards, but these do not exempt a student from all personal responsibility. For example, for students with a mood disorder, having a schedule with minimal sleep disruption may be important and may require the trainee to be given a schedule whereby overnight call responsibilities are minimised. However, since medical training requires being able to care for patients overnight, 'reasonable accommodations' could not be expected to preclude all overnight call responsibilities.

If a trainee is not able to take overnight calls, he or she could be dismissed because of not being able to manage their core professional responsibilities. Besides, the way in which medical students are evaluated is based on their behaviours, not on medical or psychiatric diagnoses. Once accommodations have been made that the school considers reasonable, the student should be able to successfully complete all requirements of the programme, just like any other medical student. While behaviours deemed inappropriate or unprofessional cannot be excused by disability, a situation such as this needs careful managing. For instance, whether, when and how the presence of such disorders and the behaviours related to them should be communicated to others requires full and careful consideration (e.g. in the case of a programme hiring such an individual). Under US law, confidential information about a student's medical diagnosis and treatment cannot be transmitted without the student's consent.[11] However, information about whether students complete their course of study without having taken any medical leave is not similarly protected.

The Association of American Medical Colleges (AAMC) recommends that any leave of absence that the student takes during education and training should be included in the MSPE or the Dean's Letter.[12] This recommendation is not mandated, and a school may or may not comply with the recommendation; however, students may be asked to explain any gaps in their medical education when they submit applications for residency programmes. Decisions about notification are best managed within the context of a conversation with the student; engaging a student in this type of conversation allows him or her to acknowledge an illness and any unprofessional behaviours that may have resulted. It is then easier to discuss the disability with future employers and to develop a plan to manage any professional challenges that the trainee faces as a consequence of having suffered a mental illness.

Trainees who are able to engage fully in this planning process should have a good chance of being able to manage these challenges successfully. It is important to remember that stealing an ultrasound machine and the resulting disciplinary proceedings are definitely reportable under the terms of the MSPE or the Dean's Letter. It is only because in this case it was felt to be a result of the student's illness and because the student eventually chose to get help that the committee did not go on to report it. Medical licensing forms that the student has to fill out for the rest of his or her career are likely to ask about treatment for mental health issues, which is why engaging the student in this conversation is so crucial.

However, AAMC suggestions about disclosing medical or administrative leaves and HIPAA (Health Insurance Portability and Accountability Act of 1996) regulations about the confidentiality of medical records are somewhat at odds when a medical disorder causes unprofessional behaviour, which makes the handling of such cases that much more difficult. While there can be a blurring of the boundaries, behaviours should generally be disclosed but not medical diagnoses.*

Summary

- Unprofessional behaviour may occur due to someone having a mental disorder; committees adjudicating unprofessional behaviour need to consider this possibility as part of their deliberations.
- The way in which this case was managed led to a 'successful' outcome, but not without considerable effort from those who had a decisive role to play.
- Patient safety and public protection are clearly relevant; while unlikely, the symptoms of mental disorder could recur and affect patient care, which emphasises the importance of communicating information about past behaviours to a future employer.
- Students with medical disorders must learn to manage their professional responsibilities when their illness is active; this may be especially challenging when the medical disorder takes the form of a psychiatric illness. For the institution handling a difficult case there is always a learning curve, especially when the case involves psychiatric illness.
- Mental illness can be causative of poor conduct; committees should be aware of this possibility but not overreact to intimidating information

---

* For classroom purposes, it may be useful to split a group of trainees in half, giving the case as written to one half of the group to consider and provide feedback on, while asking the other half to consider a variation of the case, whereby instead of there being a situation involving mental illness, the student is motivated into committing theft by adhering to 'Robin Hood' ideals; he wants to remove the equipment from a well-funded university hospital, which could recover the loss against insurance, and take it to a remote rural hospital in Africa that would have no chance of being able to afford to buy such equipment and where it could potentially benefit a significant number of women.

requests from lawyers. Protocol should be clear to help faculty handle tough cases and determine whether, when and how to alert others of problems being encountered by a trainee.

- For a licensed physician, if he or she is unable to practise because of a medical disorder, the regulator needs to be involved; in the case of medical students and trainees, the principles remain the same even if the procedures and protocols will differ.

- The AAMC provides guidance in formulating the content of a Dean's Letter – for example, regarding the disclosure of leaves of absence taken during medical school. Abiding by US (HIPAA) laws as regards the confidentiality of health records must be taken into account when it comes to notifying others such as state licensing authorities.

REFERENCES

1. www.mpts-uk.org/
2. In Brief. UK illegal drug classification. Available at: www.inbrief.co.uk/offences/drug-classification.htm (accessed 13 May 2013).
3. General Medical Council. What do you expect from a doctor outside medicine? Available at: www.gmc-uk.org/guidance/10778.asp (accessed 10 May 2013).
4. Home Office. Alcohol and drugs. Available at: www.homeoffice.gov.uk/drugs/ (accessed 13 May 2012).
5. Medicines Act 1968. Available at: www.legislation.gov.uk/ukpga/1968/67/contents#top (accessed 13 May 2013).
6. Malloch K, Porter-O'Grady P. *Introduction to Evidenced-Based Practice in Nursing and Health Care.* Burlington, MA: Jones and Bartlett; 2010.
7. Samanta A. Medical experts, the law and professional regulation. *J R Soc Med.* 2006; 99(5): 217–18.
8. Accreditation Council for Graduate Medical Education. *Program Requirements for Graduate Medical Education: psychosomatic medicine.* IV.A.2.b).(13). Chicago: ACGME; 2013. Available at: www.acgme.org/acgmeweb/Portals/0/PFAssets/ProgramRequirements/409_psychosomatic_med_psych_06012013_1-YR.pdf (accessed 6 June 2013).
9. *Regents of the University of Michigan v. Ewing.* 474 U.S. 214; 1985.
10. General Medical Council. *Duties of a Doctor.* London: GMC; 2013. Available at: www.gmc-uk.org/guidance/good_medical_practice/duties_of_a_doctor.asp (accessed 6 June 2013).
11. United States Department of Health and Human Services. *Summary of the HIPAA Privacy Rule.* Washington, DC: US Government Office for Civil Rights; 2003. Available at: www.hhs.gov/ocr/privacy/hipaa/understanding/summary/privacysummary.pdf (accessed 7 February 2013).
12. Association of American Medical Colleges. *A Guide to the Preparation of the Medical Student Performance Evaluation.* Washington, DC: AAMC; 2010. Available at: www.aamc.org/download/64496/data/mspeguide.pdf (accessed 7 February 2013).

CHAPTER 7

Australia and New Zealand

CASE STUDIES 16–29

CASE 16

A medical student is reported by his peers to be a poor team-worker.

Outline

JB, a 20-year-old male medical student, first comes to the medical school's attention in the early part of the clinical course. Three women students meet with the senior administration to say that they think JB's behaviour is inappropriate. One has witnessed JB being overfamiliar with a nurse on the ward, and two have heard him boasting in the hospital elevators about weekend sexual 'achievements'. At this point they do not wish anything to be done but they feel that they want to inform someone 'in authority'. However, they make it clear that if the matter is taken further, they do not want their names used in any investigation.

At this point, the Office of Student Affairs notes the anonymous concern in a confidential file. A few months later, a male student meets with the senior administration to represent the concerns of a group of students. They have two major worries. The first issue he reports is that a female student has described receiving inappropriate sexual advances from JB; JB had been seductive and intimidating, and the female, while refusing his advances, felt threatened. Nonetheless, she did not want to make any complaint for fear of retribution. The second issue, that the whole group of students has discussed, is the lack of involvement from JB in any group activities, as well as his frequent absences. They are puzzled as to why the medical school has not picked up on the attendance issues.

Around this same time a course convener fails JB for a clinical rotation based on his performance on the wards, his poor attendance and his tardiness in reporting for his final assessment. JB goes on to fail a written examination and is seen by the Office of Student Affairs. The failure and attendance issues are discussed, but no comment is made regarding the sexually inappropriate behaviour, as the students affected remain unwilling to be named in any complaint.

It becomes apparent at interview that JB has significant personal difficulties; he feels isolated from his peers and he is highly ambivalent about pursuing medicine as a career. He is extremely anxious when being interviewed and admits to having a social phobia. It is suggested at this stage that he see a psychiatrist for an assessment and to consider ongoing help as necessary. A break in training is also discussed while he considers personal issues, including his health and the question of his future career. Following this discussion, JB decides to take a year out and ultimately decides to withdraw from the course.

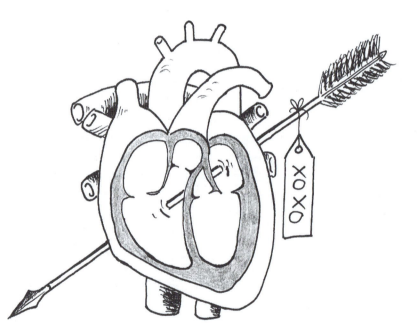

Questions

- Should or could the school have acted sooner with respect to JB's reported sexualised behaviour?
- JB was probably in agreement that he was pursuing the wrong career; how could this have been picked up sooner or, better still, when it came to selection?

- (How) can the role of student 'whistle-blower' be better acknowledged and protected?

Discussion

This young man had severe personality problems, together with heightened anxiety and issues around social avoidance. Unfortunately, his problems were not picked up early in the course, only becoming apparent through student reports and his failure in later parts of the course. The sexually inappropriate behaviour was never addressed. Initially, reports about JB were of relatively minor concern, but they escalated when his behaviour appeared predatory and threatening to a fellow student. Nonetheless, the school felt unable to act at the time because the complainant did not wish to be identified. These problems ultimately interfered with JB's performance, to the point where he withdrew from the course.

On reflection, this was a troubled student who was probably not suited to a career in medicine. As is often the case, personality problems are both difficult to identify and difficult to deal with. In this situation the sexually inappropriate behaviour was especially worrying and could easily have escalated. In retrospect, his attendance problems were related to his personality issues, social phobia and ambivalence about medicine. Worryingly, not only did the university fail to spot this early on but also it took fellow students to bring these matters to the school's attention.

This case illustrates the role fellow students can play in identifying problems, and it also highlights tensions that students can face when reporting their concerns. They are often in a good place to identify such concerns; some students can put on an appropriate 'face' when observed by staff but are less able to maintain this all the time. Furthermore, behaviours between students could be markers of how such students will behave towards future patients, by reflecting a problem with underlying attitudes. Students are good sources of information but they sometimes find it difficult to pass this on.

Cases such as this prompted the school to develop a critical incident reporting mechanism, where lapses in professional behaviour or examples of meritorious professional behaviour are now recorded and submitted to the senior administration. As part of this initiative, the school sought to draw a distinction between anonymous reporting and confidential reports. Anonymous reporting was to be discouraged; instead, the emphasis was to be put on confidentiality, which is not the same thing.

In other words, any report has to be signed by the informant, but his or her identity would not be made known to the student in question without the informant's consent. One-off reports may not be sufficient to prompt action, but if a sufficient body of evidence is acquired whereby action and/or further investigation is evidently needed, then the collective nature of the concern not only helps present a case for action but also protects the identity and vulnerability of the informant.

Summary

- Fellow students can be good informants on professional behaviours, but the reporting of concerns has its own challenges.
- The outcome was probably fair from JB's point of view; however, other students may feel let down by the school's slow response.
- Had this gone on for longer, patients and members of the public might have been put at risk.
- Critical incident reports have an important place in the toolbox of methods available to a school for detecting lapses in professionalism; staff and students need to be aware of how these systems work.
- At the time, lack of protocol in the area of critical incident reporting played a part in this case; however, lessons were learned and the chances of a similar case arising in the future were thereby diminished.
- There is little for a regulator to do in a case such as this.
- Guidelines need to be clearly written and available when needed; at the early stage of this case, neither of these conditions seemed to apply.

CASE 17

A medical student shows poor performance in doing clinical rotations.

Outline

FH is a 28-year-old final-year medical student who came to the attention of the Medical School Professionalism Committee (MSPC) the previous year. The referring clinician noted a lack of self-appraisal and self-care and a failure to recognise the need to seek appropriate mental healthcare and other medical help. FH was making poor academic progress, which she attributed to recurrence of a depressive illness, although it had been some time since she took any action in this regard. The MSPC uncovered a history of depression, and although FH had seen her general practitioner (GP), she had no contact with her psychiatrist during the entire medical programme. While this may have been suggestive of an improvement, previously she had been advised as to the importance of keeping in regular contact with both her GP and her psychiatrist. At present, her clinical teachers are unaware of this vulnerability.

A new referral is made to the MSPC, which this time refers to 'vague behaviour, lack of awareness of timetables and responsibilities, poor attendance at compulsory activities, and poor participation.' In addition, there is a contemporaneous report from another clinician indicating a degree of dishevel-ment in her appearance. This time, FH rationalises the complaints by reference to financial difficulties relating to the winding up of a loan. She also cites a lack of proper mentorship at the hospital where she is based. In response to questioning, FH admits that she has not kept up regular attendance with her psychiatrist, although from time to time she did see her GP. During the interview she says that things are improving and that she is now focused on completing the programme. Again, FH is advised to maintain regular medical contact, and to be more active in requesting feedback from her tutors.

Later in the year, a third referral to the MSPC takes place, prompted by obser-vations of suspicious behaviour in relation to drug misuse, although these suspicions are unsubstantiated. At about this time, FH abjectly fails an objec-tive structured clinical examination (OSCE), with several different examiners commenting that they are concerned about her poor performance given her late stage in the programme. FH is interviewed by a number of senior academics and the previous advice is reiterated. A pattern is emerging, with this student having being referred to the MSPC three times.

This same year FH is reported to have forged consultant physician pre-scriptions for hypnotics at one of the teaching hospitals and to have stolen benzodiazepine ampoules from another. She is promptly called in to see the senior administration; on questioning, FH rationalises her actions as 'treatment for her medical conditions'. At the hospital's request, police become involved, and the medical school excludes FH from the programme. The university in turn notifies the Medical Board of Australia (MBA) of these events, which con-ducts its own investigation, concluding that FH's fitness to practise is impaired. All medical students in Australia are registered with the MBA, and with such a ruling coming after her suspension from the medical programme this spells the end of her aspiration to become a doctor.

Questions

- To what extent are medical schools responsible for the health and welfare of their students?
- How can respect for privacy in a health matter be reconciled with the loss of 3–4 years of medical training?
- Should firmer action have been taken earlier? How likely is it that an early intervention would have avoided the eventual outcome?
- Could mandatory notification of student impairment potentially help improve the management of students *and* the protection of the public?

Discussion

The initial referral to professional committees is often in response to poor academic performance. Poor attendance is another frequent complaint that is symptomatic of other problems. Depression is relatively common among doctors and medical students, and most schools are alert to this possibility. Students cannot be forced to seek medical treatment, but schools have a measure of responsibility in advising students of the benefits of receiving appropriate treatment. A further question is how much a school should monitor student compliance when advice has been given. There are logistic and ethical boundary limitations to mounting an overt attempt to see if the student is following up and keeping her medical appointments. FH is entitled to her privacy and medical confidentiality. At the same time, a school needs to know when to act; these issues have to be dealt with appropriately and with some sensitivity.

The second referral and FH's evasive rationalisation illustrate how complex and difficult the interpretation of behaviours can be when reflective of an underlying mental health condition. The interaction of personal difficulties, a mental disorder of unknown contemporary clinical severity, the different personalities and expectations of staff involved, and possibly legitimate grievances concerning inadequate teaching, all contribute to the difficulty of assessing referrals for vague behaviour and poor attendance. Such situations require patient and supportive discussion, and even then may well result in uncertainty on the part of committees. Careful monitoring is important for those responsible for overseeing this student, especially in that a previous intervention had been deemed necessary.

By the time of the third referral (for suspicious behaviour and poor academic performance), the school authorities were ready to give a rapid response, although this does not imply that making a judgement is going to be straightforward or easy. Programme and university rules impose constraints on what actions academic staff can take, including preventing a student from progressing out of concern for the student and concern for members of the public. Some universities appear reluctant to act against students unless and until some serious unlawful activity occurs; this causes one to question a school's role in protecting the public and serving the community, as opposed to looking after the interests of the university, the medical school and its students.

Criminal activities like those described in the later stages of this case, although underpinned by inadequate management of a serious mental disorder and possibly other personality and social factors, could be seen by staff as an opportunity to deal with an underperforming student. By the time these events occurred, a clear pattern had emerged, featuring mental illness, non-compliance, lack of self-awareness and self-appraisal and poor academic progress. It is perhaps surprising that FH managed to progress as far as her final year, and one of the problems for professional educators and students like FH is that such patterns take time to develop. By the time they cause real problems, students will have invested time, money and effort, only to be faced with the possibility of not graduating. In the process, a student will surely have had to relinquish other opportunities.

Medical boards and councils differ in the areas of student activity with which they are concerned. If FH did eventually graduate and go on to practise medicine, the MBA would have taken on a formal supervisory and monitoring role, which would continue into the next stage of training. Such arrangements are not uncommon, and in the case of FH it was probably only the criminal element in the later stages of her case that prevented her from graduating and continuing with her training.

Summary

- Medical students, like doctors, tend to have higher rates of mental disorders, particularly depression, than the general community, which can manifest as poor professionalism.
- The outcome for FH is far from satisfactory; however, it is difficult to provide adequate support for struggling students unless they fail an exam or commit an offence that brings them to the attention of the school.
- Schools should include student impairment in their duty-of-care commitments; while recognising limits on when an intervention can be made, schools have a duty of care to the community as well as to individual students. Being fair and supportive to a student should not be at the expense of failing in public protection, which could require exclusion from programmes, even at late stages.
- Poor medical follow-up in relation to mental health is not uncommon; in the case of medical students, it may be a question of considering what actions are needed in order to trigger an appropriate intervention by the school.
- Protocols are important in dealing with a complex interaction of student issues – educational, psychological and interpersonal – which can make interpreting and managing student behaviour and welfare fairly complex. Schools should try to ensure sensitive and skilful membership of professionalism committees and provide adequate monitoring for students.
- Medical registration authorities play an important partner role with universities in managing impaired students.
- Guidelines need to be available for staff to help them in managing students such as this.

CASE 18

A medical student gets a little too close to her patients.

Outline

MC, a 22-year-old female medical student, comes to the school's attention because of matters relating to small group work during her clinical years. She is a capable student and is doing well in her examinations; however, fellow students find her difficult to get on with, and she tends to make personal statements about other students in tutorials. Tutors report that she also tends to be overly familiar with them, intruding into their personal lives. This tendency is noted with some concern, and after MC fails one of her clinical rotations, she is called for interview with a senior administrator, whose concern is mainly about MC's professional conduct. It had also been noted that MC spent a disproportionate amount of time with a particular patient on the wards, even bringing in flowers from her own garden. The main concern here is that the patient told MC important information about her past psychiatric history; MC then kept that information from the treatment team because she felt that she had a *special* relationship with the patient.

MC is referred to the Fitness to Practise Committee, which, in consultation with the senior administration, decides to place her with a mentor, who is a senior and respected clinical member of staff. The mentor meets with the student regularly and they discuss professional boundary issues. A report from the mentor indicates that MC has made considerable progress, concluding that no further problems need to be resolved. However, senior administration decides to refer MC for some personal therapy. It appears that her loneliness and interaction style are making it difficult for her to form friendships and, as a consequence, she is using patients to meet some of her own needs.

Questions

- When do personality and social problems become matters of professionalism?
- How easy is it for medical schools to identify and support a student such as this?
- To what extent is professionalism about nature as opposed to nurture?
- Is it ever appropriate for a medical student to form a special relationship with a patient?

Discussion

This student displays problems with personal and professional boundaries. She does not know when it is appropriate to keep her thoughts to herself, when and whether private lives are a matter for public discussion, and when kindness to a patient crosses the line and becomes an undue closeness. The most serious problem, however, is not sharing relevant clinical information with other treating staff, even though the intervention turned out to be very effective. The use of a senior, respected mentor, attuned to professional boundary issues, helped MC to interpret and make sense of her clinical experiences.

This case perhaps illustrates that professionalism can sometimes be an acquired attribute. Parents, upbringing and role models all play a part, but above all, professionalism needs to be nurtured by encountering and mastering difficult situations, preferably with help from sympathetic and supportive members of staff. Professionalism sometimes needs time, space and opportunity to develop. Just as learning can occur best after a mistake has been made if there is an opportunity to reflect on and learn from the event, professionalism is a skill that can improve with time as a trainee learns to respond to challenging, complex situations. In other words, professionalism has elements of both nature *and* nurture.

Occasionally, the stress of a situation builds to a point where a trainee displays less than professional behaviour. Given the right circumstances and enough pressure, any individual may be at risk of displaying less than ideal professional behaviours. However, most people have sufficient insight to be able to recognise that when challenging situations arise, they need to develop coping strategies and to seek out the necessary support. It has been found in other settings that professional boundary issues are more likely to arise when there is a lack of balance in personal relationships.[1] In this case, gentle feedback with help and support from a mentor seemed sufficient to ensure a successful outcome.

Summary

- Learning appropriate boundaries in the doctor–patient relationship and interpersonal relationships is an important element of professionalism.
- Some problems with boundaries only come to light after exposure to relevant clinical experiences when a student is nearing the end of the course; overall, the outcome of this case seems fair and just.
- Keeping relevant information from the clinical team could have endangered a patient, which highlights the importance of establishing personal boundaries with patients.
- Ongoing, direct supervision was important for this student, meaning that clinical tutors need to be well trained and at hand.
- There were no protocol issues in this case.
- Concerns in this case did not need to be brought to the attention of the regulator.
- Lack of balance in personal relationships cannot be covered by guidelines; appropriate local intervention is probably the best course of action.

CASE 19

A senior medical student shows sudden deterioration in his clinical performance.

Outline

A final-year medical student, DZ, is 6 months away from completing the pro-gramme and entering the workforce. He performs unexpectedly badly at an observed structured clinical examination, demonstrating poor interpersonal skills and clinical reasoning. Examiners record comments, using phrases such as 'abrupt with patients', 'haphazard history taking', 'muddled thinking', and 'unable to define appropriate differential diagnoses'. However, DZ had com-fortably passed a multiple-choice question paper the previous week, and in previous years he had always performed in the middle of the cohort. The Board of Examiners, nonetheless, recommends a 'fail' decision, and the student is invited to meet with the year convener, Dr C, to discuss this unexpected result.

DZ explains that he has a chronic mental illness that is normally under con-trol, but that recently he ceased taking his medication. This is because he has been feeling well and does not want to have to carry on taking medication for the rest of his life. He had not previously told the school about the illness and had not accessed student support, explaining that 'it was nobody else's busi-ness'. He complains that the 'fail' decision is unfair.

DZ had kept these things entirely to himself, prompting Dr C to write to DZ asking for an explanation as to why he did not self-disclose. At the same time, Dr C emails the director of academic studies, explaining the situation that has arisen. Dr C tries to find clarification on the issue but comes up against a complete lack of guidance. The school argues that in the absence of disclosure and with no previous signs of erratic behaviour or performance, they had no reason to suspect any mental illness.

DZ decides to lodge a formal appeal against his grade, which, he argues, only came about because of his having a long-term underlying mental health condition. In law, this would be classed as a disability, bringing into questions potential issues of unfair discrimination. In lodging his appeal DZ is assisted by a lawyer who also happens to be a relative. The final decision goes in favour of the school, upholding the previous decision. The head of school notifies the Australian Health Practitioner Regulation Agency on the grounds that the student might decide to cease medication again in the future and suffer deterio-rating performance, thereby putting patients at risk. The student is told about the notification; the family threatens to sue for breach of confidentiality but it does not follow through.

Questions

- To what extent should current poor performance in a clinical examination be compensated for by past strong performance?
- To what extent is this about managing a disability, and when does a disability become an impairment in terms of professionalism?
- What responsibilities do students with disabilities have, and to whom?
- Was notifying the regulatory agency necessary and appropriate?

Discussion

Australian medical students are required to register with their local medical board, and students with potential impairments are encouraged to self-report in order to initiate appropriate support and health assessments prior to commencing work. Mandatory reporting requirements exist for students having either a criminal conviction, or a potential impairment to safe practice. While there is every reason to act to promote public safety, this puts the medical school in an awkward situation.

The situation may warrant mandatory notification prior to graduation, but such action could be seen as a breaching of medical confidentiality, and, in any case, the threshold for 'impairment' is not well defined. The question of thresholds relating to disability and impairment is primarily one of law and public policy. While resources for this topic are not easily found, the Higher Education Occupational Physicians/Practitioners Society has published useful guidance.[2] In this case, the head of school made the notification, knowing that the information would be filed by the regulator and acted on only when the individual applied for medical registration. It is to be expected that DZ would have to pass a health assessment before being deemed well enough to practise.

It is not for the person with the mental health condition to decide whether or not the impairment is important – that judgement has to be made by others. It is difficult to be objective in such a situation; nonetheless, sensitive information should be treated by the school with due respect to medical confidentiality. While the issue of confidentiality did not result in legal action in this case, it would be wise for schools to seek legal advice on reporting policy, including how and when it should be applied. Rights of the public to be protected from a doctor who is 'unsafe' can trump individual rights to privacy of information, and on that basis a regulator needs to know. The greatest difficulty is knowing what the school or regulator needs to know without first having to invade student privacy.

Reporting requirements would not be effective if they resulted in students withholding important information about their health. If a medical student finds him-or herself in a tight spot, citing human rights violation as a defence could possibly be justified; however, if students do not meet their obligation to disclose relevant information in a timely way, such a defence may do little other than to buy time. DZ should have disclosed his medical condition sooner; his failure to do so destroyed his own defence, which could well be a reason why the case against the school was not pursued. Rights and obligations go hand in hand, and while public protection is sometimes in conflict with the right to privacy and freedom from discrimination, individual cases can only be judged on their merits.

Summary

- Failure to disclose information that might impact on one's ability to perform is unethical and unprofessional.
- The appeal is opportunistic on account of DZ's failure to accept responsibility for his illness, and the school probably did nothing wrong; on this basis the outcome does seem fair and appropriate.
- Public safety is important when it comes to doctors having a mental illness; it should not preclude them from working. However, if DZ has patient responsibilities when he decides to stop medication, there will always be issues around safety.
- There do not seem to be any failings here on the part of the school, and from an internal point of view, there are no obvious lessons to be learned.
- No issues around protocol arise with this case.
- Because of coming up against a lack of clarity in public policy and the law, there is scope for better guidance to be made available to schools to help them handle difficult cases. This issue would best be addressed in consultation with the regulator.
- Lack of guidance is a relevant factor in this case, and the issue of when a disability becomes an impairment needs to be made clear.

CASE 20

A medical student displays poor attitudes towards women.

Outline

MW, a 22-year-old male international medical student, comes from a country where traditionally men have a more dominant place in society than women. His interactions with men are congenial, and his academic progress, while not stellar, is generally satisfactory. However, there have been tensions between him and some of his female small group classmates, and during a tutorial one of his female classmates challenges his views relating to the suggested management of a case. He becomes angry at the disagreement and hits her, and while no physical injury is caused, the classmate is very shaken, and the incident is reported to the dean, who in turn notifies the university proctor.

The case is eventually referred to the Fitness to Practise Committee, and MW is given a warning to the effect that a repeat incident will result in expulsion. He accepts this warning but appears to show no remorse. The remainder of the year proceeds without any incidents. The following year, MW is required to write up a case report on a patient based in the community. It becomes apparent that the report provided is of a patient he had never seen; when this indiscretion is brought to his attention, he denies the dishonesty until presented with irrefutable evidence; at this point, he admits that he had falsified the report. This falsification meets with the university's definitions of dishonest practice. His situation is again brought to the university's Fitness to Practise Committee, and they recommend that in light of the previous incident and warning, he should be expelled. The university upholds this decision, and despite MW having completed over 5 years of study in medicine and passing all academic requirements, he is expelled and leaves with no formal qualifications.

Questions

- Both incidents were about professional standards; however, they were not of the same nature; was this important?
- How do these 'offences' compare with each other, and who needs to know?
- Did cultural conditioning affect MW's ability to function as a trainee, and if so, what are the implications?

Discussion

MW acted unprofessionally on two separate occasions, and while the two breaches were of a different nature, the university took the view that together they reflected a standard of unprofessionalism that was unacceptable. His behaviour was made worse by the fact that he showed no remorse for the violent incident and that he denied dishonesty in his case report. These were two separate incidents rather than repeated behaviours, and a question that needs asking is whether there were any mitigating factors. It could be argued that the warning after the first incident applied narrowly to a repeat of a similar incident – in other words, the second incident would also have had to involve physical assault in order for him to be expelled. However, the university chose to apply a wider interpretation, questioning MW's character and lack of professionalism.

Relevant to this case were cultural differences between New Zealand and his home county, where being challenged by a female classmate might have been regarded as sufficient justification for violent behaviour. Therefore, the question has to be asked as to whether standards set by the home institution should apply, or rules and cultural mores pertaining to the student's home country? The university rightly took the view that the cultural expectations of New Zealand mattered most, and ethical and legal frameworks of the country where MW was doing his training were indeed paramount. While the two incidents were different, the university took the view that together they represented an unacceptable pattern of behaviour and that MW was not fit to practise medicine.

The next thing to consider was whether or not police should have been involved, and given that carrying out a physical assault is indeed a crime, the answer is probably 'yes'. A university proctor has 'campus police' duties, and in theory it was for the proctor to decide whether or not to inform the police. There do not seem to be any good reasons for keeping the incident of violence from the police other than to avoid escalation.

Summary

- Cultural differences among students need to be acknowledged, when and where appropriate, but they do not provide an excuse for unprofessional behaviours, especially if they feature acts of violence or blatant dishonesty.
- While in some respects the outcome was fair and proportionate, it did not take into account that the two one-off breaches of professional conduct were of a different nature; MW could have won on appeal.
- The university had to decide whether or not to involve the police, and in making that judgement, the university needed to be mindful of its public responsibility.
- It is not unusual for medical schools to encounter students who are generally competent but who nonetheless give cause for concern for non-academic reasons; each case can only be assessed on its merits.
- Following protocol means a higher chance of success in the event of a legal challenge; MW chose not to take that route, but institutions have to consider whether or not they could defend their actions in court; acting in the public interest may be insufficient as a defence if a serious injustice is committed.
- This case was not one for the regulator.
- Guidelines generally help if they are well written and up to date; in this case national guidelines helped inform a disciplinary decision made at local level.

CASE 21

A medical student has a pattern of absences and unreliability.

Outline

AB is a 23-year-old medical student in his final year. His progress in the earlier part of the course was uneventful; during later years in clinical settings, staff know him as being a pleasant and somewhat charming young man. There are times when he is noted as being absent without any clear explanation, but somehow he always seems to be present at times when tutors are likely to notice his presence.

When he asks for brief periods of leave during the course, his reasons are always plausible, but they occur slightly too frequently. It is also noted that he is overly casual in his manner with patients and nurses, and they comment that he appears somewhat indifferent. In the final year, as he is given more clinical responsibility, two critical events take place. First, he claims to have taken blood off a patient and sent it to the lab, but it turns out later that he had not. Second, he reports that he had examined a patient when he had not. These markers of reliability and honesty concern his supervisors, who bring his case to the attention of the Medical Student Progress Committee. In discussion, more issues come to light around his apparent unreliability, his lack of punctuality, and the charming manner in which he explains away issues when confronted.

Upon questioning from the senior administration officials, AB makes it clear that he thinks everyone is making a fuss about nothing. Nevertheless, because of concerns about professionalism and his lack of response to constructive feedback, he fails to pass the year. He accepts the offer of a mentor and when he repeats the year, he manages to complete the course satisfactorily.

Questions

- Lapses in professionalism may seem less serious if someone always responds in a manner that is charming and polite; when do you draw the line and say 'enough is enough'?
- AB's lack of attention and unprofessional conduct is troubling, but was it right that he had to resit the year?
- Should the university have picked this up sooner, and did it do its job in sorting the matter prior to graduation?

Discussion

Interestingly, there was little to cause concern during the early part of training; however, the two episodes in his final year were sufficient to trigger concerns about professionalism and prevent him from passing the year. In retrospect, there were markers all along. There were avoidance behaviours, and he developed a coping strategy of being around just enough to satisfy tutors but not necessarily enough to satisfy requirements for his learning. AB also illustrates the effect of 'charm', whereby someone with natural ability and charisma can get away with behaviours that others might not.

Some problems with professionalism only come to light when a student is given clinical responsibility and is under close observation. Almost by definition, such situations arise in the later parts of the course. Systems may not be sensitive enough to detect issues when they arise early in the course. In this case the more likely explanation is that issues did not come to light because the situations in which this student was placed required different skills from those needed earlier in the course.

This student declined the offer of a mentor. Not all help that is offered needs to be taken up, and it could be argued that if a student passes the course without extra help, then the right decisions have been made. However, in retrospect, one could arrive at an alternative point of view. Provision of a mentor may be 'therapeutic', but from a medical school perspective, it could also be seen as 'diagnostic'.

In other words, a mentor may not just help the student; a mentor may also help the medical school understand how, if at all, student attitudes may be changing. This dual role of a mentor (therapeutic and diagnostic) needs to be made explicit, lest the trust implicit in the mentor–student relationship becomes ambiguous. The fact that AB passed the year does not necessarily mean that the student's professional attitudes have changed, as he may have simply learned to display the right behaviours at the right times and to the right people.

Those involved in the case wondered if there was a place for *mandating* a mentor in instances such as this, to help both the student and the school. If this had been done, perhaps the appointed person would not be called a mentor but would instead be given a more descriptive name, such as a 'personal tutor' or 'supervisor'. What is of most concern in this case is the student's lack of concern over issues of reliability, responsibility and respect for patients and staff, plus a general lack of empathy that did not come to light until late in the course. In retrospect, this could have been picked up earlier by peer and/ or multisource feedback. While the student ultimately did graduate, concerns remained as to whether or not there had been significant change in his underlying attitudes and behaviours.

Summary

- Some problems with professionalism only come to light later in the course; professional behaviours are dependent on context and may only become apparent when a person is under pressure.
- Professionalism is not necessarily innate, and nor is it suddenly acquired;

instead, it develops over time, often as a result of being placed in increasingly challenging situations; there is no suggestion here that the student was treated unfairly.

- Having the time and space to reflect on challenging situations helps with professional development; however, some personal aspects of professional values are present long before medical school; in this case, the student did not appear concerned about dishonesty or putting patients at risk.
- A personal supervisor or mentor may assist not only in helping a student but also in helping a medical school understand how or when professional attitudes may be changing.
- The relationship between attitudes and behaviours is potentially complex; the latter may be easier to remediate than the former, and it is not easy to devise protocols that are sensitive to this difference.
- This case need not concern the regulator.
- While guidelines usually help, they need to be sufficiently sensitive to deal with the complexity of underlying issues.

CASE 22

A medical student, repeating an academic year, is taking shortcuts.

Outline

SD is repeating the second year of medical school; he failed the previous year after failing to comply with requirements of the programme. He maintains that failing year two was unfair and he resents having to repeat the year. Now, he has unsatisfactory attendance at compulsory small group tutorials and is referred to the professionalism committee. Just before the interview, the committee receives two further independent reports, one indicating that his long-case report shows marked similarities with that submitted by another student, and the other indicating that he submitted three clinical cases that had been signed off by his uncle. The uncle is a consultant at another teaching hospital within the school's network, but he is not the clinical preceptor and, according to course rules, only the preceptor is authorised to sign off. The committee thus has three separate issues to consider.

SD argues to the committee that attendance at the small group sessions is a waste of time, as he finds the format unproductive; also, he finds it boring going over the same material for the second time. Regarding the plagiarism issue, SD states that collaborating with a peer on the final case is simply how things work, and he considers that presenting a significant amount of common written work is fully justified. Regarding his clinical case reports, SD sees no problem with the fact that his uncle assessed his work, as he is a prominent physician and could obviously assess SD's competence in basic history-taking and physical examination. SD backs this up by asserting that his uncle is highly professional, saying he was unaware that the medical programme only allowed the preceptor to sign off on clinical work.

The committee forms the view that SD has transgressed in all three areas. First, SD fails to attend compulsory tutorial sessions, which is a straightforward case of breaking publicised programme rules. Second, while the structure of clinical assessments allows two students to see patients together, there is a clear direction that case presentations are to be independently prepared, and so the plagiarism allegation is also upheld. Third, the committee considers that having his uncle sign off is unacceptable conduct on the part of SD; clear directions were given to students concerning appropriate assessors for their work, and the committee forms the view that the uncle had himself behaved unprofessionally.

The views of the committee are conveyed clearly and strongly to SD, on the basis that such feedback should help him to see that his behaviour is not in the interests of peers or patients, and also not in his own interest as a student wishing to progress and graduate. Following the interview, committee members share their exasperation at SD's apparent lack of insight into why the committee stated that he should consider himself responsible in relation to the matters discussed. They were unsure as to whether or not to communicate with SD's uncle and express their concerns. It is likely that SD will eventually graduate, although at this stage it is not known.

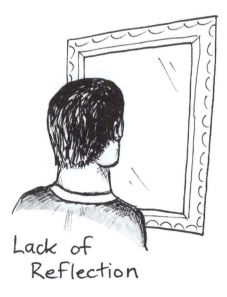

Lack of
Reflection

Questions

- Should medical school admissions procedures include screening for personality factors, and if so, how?
- To what extent should medical schools consider themselves potential educators in relation to other members of the profession (e.g. SD's uncle), who the school perceives as having behaved inappropriately?
- To what extent should medical schools make allowance for learning preferences of individual students?
- To what extent should repeating students be permitted to pick and choose what they attend during a repeat year?
- Should SD's uncle be contacted, and should he be part of the remediation plan?

Discussion

SD is an aggrieved and resentful student. He is aware that his failures could probably have been avoided, but there are limits as to his degree of insight. He established a pattern over time, during his repeated year and the prior year, continuing to challenge different aspects of the programme. His perception of group sessions as being unproductive and boring belie a self-centredness about group work rather than an approach that values mutual learning, as well as false confidence in his mastery of the course material.

Both the plagiarism issue and the signing-off issue suggest that SD has not taken the trouble, even during his second attempt at year two, to familiarise himself with the programme rules. He should have known that medical schools usually do not allow 'partial' repeat years, but in any case, this should have been discussed and clarified prior to commencing the repeat year. This may suggest laziness, unjustified confidence, arrogance or a combination of all three. The nature of SD's motivation to study and practise medicine could also be called into question.

The patterns established by this stage point to there being more than one underlying problem. As in many cases of poor student performance (and poor performance of qualified practitioners), the possibility of mental illness must be entertained, if only to be excluded later. In this case, it is likely that an attitudinal schema or particular personality style underpins SD's approach, which could be problematic for the student, medical educators, the medical profession and, ultimately, for patients. SD could continue to avoid rules and requirements in clinical practice, ignore feedback or fail to seek it and be resentful of any setbacks or criticism later on.

The signing-off of SD's clinical cases by his uncle presents a different problem, but one that is also likely to be underpinned by attitudinal factors. Both student and practitioner fail to be aware of appropriate boundaries, and while

SD had formal instruction concerning boundary issues in medical practice, this has apparently not been effective (or else he was absent from the lecture). However, greater fault perhaps lies with the uncle, who fails to avoid a conflict of interest. He blurs a boundary that exists to ensure objectivity in gauging student performance and displays disregard not just for the boundaries but also for standards of professionalism in medical education. While the school has no jurisdiction over the uncle, if they were so minded, they could bring the matter to the attention of others, such as an employer or regulator.

Summary

- Student personalities and attitudes characterised by arrogance, excess confidence, lack of insight and resentfulness are not good for patients or the future career of doctors. Unprofessionalism in this case is not limited to the conduct of the medical student; professionalism rules are equally applicable to students and practising professionals, even though the practical implications differ when it comes to enforcement.
- It was entirely appropriate for SD to be reprimanded for lack of professionalism; it is his responsibility to know about and adhere to the rules.
- Patient safety issues do not arise in this case; however, attitudes that persist over time could lead to difficulties later on.
- Medical schools have an obligation from time to time to take action in relation to people for whom they are not directly responsible, but whose behaviour affects the welfare of the school. Education and training in medicine does not take place in isolation; it regularly extends beyond the boundaries of an institution.
- Programme rules are linked to academic progress, and medical schools should apply them rigorously and consistently. Protocol was properly followed in this case.
- As it happened, the case did not involve the regulator.
- Medical programmes must develop and publish unambiguous programme rules, together with relevant sanctions, that students should adhere to in order to ensure adequate performance and equity across the student body.

CASE 23

A medical student is having a relationship with an administrative member of staff.

Outline

BJ, a 24-year-old male, third-year graduate entry medical student is noticed to be in a relationship with SM, a 23-year-old administration officer in the assessment office. It seems to be a happy circumstance for both, and the two often have lunch together in the hospital café. BJ often drops into her office to say hello and to discuss plans for later in the day. SM's colleagues become concerned because she has access to both examination paper results and data relating to BJ's class, which sit on a computer in her office. While most of her colleagues believe that the relationship is genuine, some fellow students are spreading rumours that this is a subterfuge to allow BJ to get prior knowledge of examination questions.

BJ does better than expected on the next set of written exams; the head of the examinations office, who is aware of the relationship and has already told SM to be careful, feels that while she has no evidence with which to confront SM, someone ought to investigate. She informs the head of school of her concerns, who then asks a senior member of staff to speak to both parties and report back. By this stage there are more rumours floating among the student body, especially in year three.

Informal inquiries reveal no actionable wrongdoing, but the head of school, mindful of the sensitivity of this matter, asks the human resources department for guidance and promises to the student representative that there will be further investigations. BJ is asked to write a formal statement and told to submit it to the chair of the conduct committee, who takes the view that in the legal sense there appears to be no 'case to answer'. However, some action needs to be taken in order to assure credibility in the examinations process. BJ is eventually asked to reconsider the relationship or to seek to transfer his studies to another institution; he is assured of good references. Meanwhile, SM is given a written warning and told that if any wrongdoing is subsequently proven, it could cost her job. BJ protests, and argues that his human rights are being infringed by being asked to make this choice. SM, who is frightened by the written warning, decides to end the relationship. BJ is furious and says he plans to take action against the school.

Questions

- How appropriate is a relationship between a student and a staff member? How would such a judgement be made?
- How fair is it to respond to student gossip without solid evidence?
- How might the school have managed this situation better?

Discussion

This case sounds some alarms; the relationship itself is not 'inappropriate' in the way that it would be if a relationship arose between a student and a patient. However, SM's position is not very tenable, having potentially conflicting loyalties. No laws are being broken, and there is no suggestion that the relationship is anything other than genuine; however, doing nothing on the part of the medical school might not be an option, given the accusations that have arisen. It is unlikely that either the school or the university would have specific guidance relating to such matters, although the university would have a general policy on conflict of interest.

If everyone does as they should and SM is able to keep her work entirely separate from her relationship, then there need not be any difficulties, especially if BJ stops dropping by the office. However, because of the exam result, both parties are now under suspicion. In terms of investigation it is always difficult to prove a negative – that is, it is easier to prove an action than a non-action, and once rumours begin they tend not to go away. From the school's perspective, if the integrity of the examination process is in question, the consequences could be quite far-reaching. A situation that before was only mildly challenging then becomes more serious.

The burden of proof of wrongdoing is on a third party (i.e. the medical school); without proof, BJ should not have been asked to make choices between remaining at the medical school or maintaining this relationship. SM's desire to try to keep her job is perfectly understandable. While it is a matter of opinion as to how the case could have been handled better, there is potential for a legal case deriving from BJ's allegations of human rights infringement. Relationships are personal, but the circumstances in which they take place may not be, and where there is a 'community' involvement, as in this case, then it may be justified for someone in authority to 'intervene'. How to intervene is the hard part.

The ultimatum given to BJ lies at the margins of acceptability. The outcome seems unfair, but one can neither control human relationships nor predict human behaviour, and situations that on their own may not be very serious can quickly escalate. The relationship was most likely a bad idea from the beginning; however, raising the issue of human rights has some legitimacy, although a violation still has to be proven. In any case, a process of appeal should have been made available to BJ.

There are no patient safety issues, but public interest is involved in this case because the exam system has to be seen to be robust and credible, and the interests of the student body have to be taken into account. Guidelines from the United Kingdom give advice on working with colleagues and on relationships with patients,[3,4] but not on relationships between students and administrators. Very often academic leaders have to make judgements based on incomplete information in the absence of formal definitive guidance. Each case has unique elements and this is no exception; the best result may simply be to try to achieve the 'least worst' outcome.

Summary

- This cases raises a range of issues from appropriateness of a relationship between a student and an administrative officer, to protecting the integrity of the examination process, respecting human rights, and a lack of clarity as regards processes and procedures.
- The case does not seem to have been handled especially well, but it is not easy to point the finger of blame at any one individual or system; the outcome does seem unfair, especially as there was no real opportunity to launch an appeal.
- Patient safety issues do not arise, but community interests are important because of the need for the school to maintain its integrity.
- Examinations are a vital part of education and training, and efforts must be made to ensure their validity.
- Failure to follow protocol was possibly less of an issue than lack of clarity as to what it actually was.
- This matter can be dealt with internally, although if not handled properly it could end up in court. This case is unlikely to be of interest to the regulator.
- Not every situation is covered by guidelines; lawyers, however, could refer more broadly to employment and/or human rights legislation.

CASE 24

A medical student has a pattern of taking leave for non-specific illnesses.

Outline

JC is a 20-year-old medical student. Prior to her clinical placements she had progressed well, but during her clinical years she develops recurrent abdominal pain that, despite extensive and prolonged investigation, has no formal diagnosis. The abdominal pain often coincides with challenging clinical activities or assessments. She frequently asks for time off, sometimes for reasons of illness, and at other times to enable her to attend investigations and/or medical appointments. Sometimes she is seen out and about by staff members when she is officially 'off sick'; outwardly she appears well. Initially members of staff involved with teaching JC were sympathetic to her requests, but when it becomes apparent that these requests are frequent and extending into each stage of the course, the school begins to be concerned. Although when present she functions at a good level, the cumulative time taken off means that she is missing large parts of the course, including assessments. These have to be made up at a later stage, at some inconvenience to the course organisers.

Before deciding whether to grant the time off, some medical staff (not involved in a treating role) want to obtain additional medical information about her illness. The situation is compounded by enough investigations being 'ambiguously abnormal' such that diagnostic clarity can never be fully achieved; suspicions are raised that the illnesses may be more reflective of anxiety and stress than anything else. JC declines to seek psychiatric help. Eventually, the medical school asks module conveners to direct any requests for time off through the administration so that a consistent approach can be taken and the cumulative effect of sick leave can be calculated.

JC ultimately has to repeat a part of the course, because too much of the year has been missed, but JC feels the medical school is being unreasonable and lacking in compassion in expecting her to make up for the missed components of the course. When seen by the senior administration she blames 'the system'; she is preoccupied by her health problems and unable to reflect on the impact of her absences. In spite of these challenges and continuing health problems, JC eventually graduates, albeit over a longer period of time than her peers. However, her case is reported to the Medical Council of New Zealand (MCNZ), which monitors her progress post graduation. She stays on to work at the same district hospital, and her postgraduate years continue to be marked by recurrent absences from work.

Questions

- Should an undiagnosed problem be treated less sympathetically than one that has a formal diagnosis?
- Can or should a medical school require a student to seek a psychiatric opinion?
- To what extent are health concerns providing a cover for her failings in professionalism?
- How should a clinical teacher define the boundary between providing teaching or pastoral support and asking personal questions in order to proffer a medical opinion?

Discussion

This case proved to be very difficult, and it illustrates some of the problems that can arise when medical school staff members are not just teachers and academics, but also practising clinicians. It can sometimes be difficult for staff to recognise where these boundaries lie, and it is easy for the teaching role of a staff member to drift into a clinical role. This becomes critically important if staff members seek medical information solely in order to help them make an academic decision. In such a situation, preserving medical confidentiality for a student can be quite challenging.

Medical schools should never allow progression based on what a student *might* be able to achieve, as opposed to what he or she actually *does* achieve; if students miss an assessment they should be given another opportunity, when well, to be able to demonstrate competence. Thus, regardless of reasons for a student being absent, especially from an assessment, each student ultimately has to be able to demonstrate competence in each clinical area. Anything short of that would be a failure of public duty on the part of the school. In this case, the medical school, following extensive discussion with relevant members of staff, decided to take a coordinated approach, which was mediated by the senior administration. However, the student perceived this as being *uncompassionate* – a criticism that strikes at the heart of how a clinician sees him- or herself; additionally, support provided by the senior administration was simply met with more complaints about the system.

The situation might have been easier to deal with had the student been failing academic components of the course. However, when well and present, she functioned at a reasonable level, eventually passing all components of the course. Although a serious adverse outcome was avoided, there is another dimension to the case that needs consideration. Under New Zealand law (the Health Practitioners Competence Assurance Act 2003), there is 'a statutory duty on any health practitioner or employer of health practitioners to notify the MCNZ if any graduating student has a health problem that would not enable them to perform the functions required for practice'. Thus, the decision was made to refer the case on to the MCNZ. This was so as to be compliant with the law and enable ongoing monitoring arrangements to be put in place post graduation.

While New Zealand law permits or requires information on health issues to be conveyed to the MCNZ, this does not apply to issues that would otherwise be classified as academic or professional. Given a level of ambiguity in this case as to how much of JC's problems were about health and how much about a failure to reflect on and understand aspects of professionalism, this case highlights an area of policy where there is real lack of clarity. JC's health concerns were sufficient for her details to be passed on to the MCNZ, but some members of staff felt that MC's problems with professionalism were not properly addressed.

In retrospect, members of staff do not think that they managed this student particularly well. She clearly struggled with 'abnormal illness behaviour', which proved difficult to address for both clinicians and teachers (and clinical teachers). In conclusion, legal constraints whereby information about health issues but not about issues with professionalism can be passed to the MCNZ may not always be to the benefit of students or the public.

Summary

- A significant problem for this student appeared to be a lack of ability to reflect on her own behaviour and professionalism as it related to her health problems.

- The student graduated, but ongoing involvement of the MCNZ means that she will never really be free from these concerns.
- While illness in a medical student affecting academic progress can give rise to problems for clinical academics, the possible impact on patients and the public always has to be considered.
- Clinicians keen to understand the nature of an illness may find it difficult wearing an 'academic hat'; their dichotomous roles can be a source of tension, recognition of which should be part of teacher training.
- Procedures within the school need to be sensitive to possible overlap between health and professionalism.
- Regulatory guidance surrounding the clinical academic's role in providing medical opinions regarding his or her student's health should be clarified.
- National guidelines reflecting the law were in some respects part of the problem, not the solution; the law appears insensitive to the distinction between health, professionalism and academic achievement.

CASE 25

A medical student talks a little too freely in the operating theatre.

Outline

A third-year medical student, TS, is referred to the Professional Conduct Committee (PCC) by the head of a clinical programme attached to the medical school. The referral indicates that 'while TS is generally OK, he unfortunately is somewhat gregarious and can overstep the boundaries of professional discourse on occasions'. Recently, this behaviour motivated a complaint by nursing staff at the hospital; the complaint was dealt with locally, with TS acknowledging the issues. However, different consultants mention this gregariousness, and eventually the matter is brought to the attention of the PCC.

At interview, TS tells the committee that the nurses' complaint resulted from a discussion between himself, another student and a surgeon during a surgical procedure in the operating room. The discussion was about a range of non-medical subjects, including politics, literature, religion and history. TS accepts that this discussion could have annoyed others in the operating room, and at the time he was told that 'his behaviour in the operating room was unacceptable and that as a student he should know his place'.

He is asked by the hospital director to sign a letter admitting that he was at fault and stating that this will not occur again, and that if it does occur again it will affect his future career. TS explains that he believes his comments in the operating room were simply part of a discussion that was not in any way meant to be offensive; there is no disputing that the discussion included a senior surgeon, as well as other students, and overall TS feels victimised, intimidated and hurt by the experience.

The committee advises TS to be discrete in future and to 'keep his antennae alert' to possible consequences of different interactions with medical and other healthcare staff. Committee members are concerned that this has apparently been a difficult experience for the student; furthermore, given that two other students were also under the direction of the surgeon and no complaints were filed against them, the committee wonders what was so inappropriate about TS's remarks. The situation is not helped by wording in the referral letter being rather vague and uninformative, with no detail about the initiating complaint.

The committee makes further inquiries, and the head of the clinical programme reveals that the gist of the nurses' complaint is 'cross-cultural', including inappropriate jokes. The head of the clinical programme agrees that it appears unfair that TS is potentially targeted for disciplinary action while nothing happens to the surgeon or the other students, who could have also been at fault. However, the head of the clinical programme also points out that there is a 'pecking order', whereby nurses would find it easier to complain about a student than about a senior surgeon. The head of programme then confers with the hospital director, who takes the matter seriously; however, the head of the clinical programme now considers that the matter ought to be 'buried'.

The PCC writes to TS, providing details of interactions with the hospital director and the head of the clinical programme. The difficulty faced by the PCC chair is that the head of the clinical programme's account of events does not fully address the committee's concerns, and the committee accepts that for TS the resulting state of affairs is unsatisfactory. However, the committee concludes that no further action needs to be taken.

Questions
- To what extent can the PCC really get to the bottom of the case?
- What does this case tell you about the underlying culture of some medical practice?
- How should TS respond in a situation over which he has little control?
- When is gregariousness a professionalism problem, and when do social interactions become a cause for concern?

Discussion
This case highlights numerous issues involving fair and efficient assessment and management of medical student behaviour. TS has been referred for interview on the basis of an alleged lapse in professionalism, but the referral is very vague, necessitating further discussion with the referrer. Even further inquiry

fails to reveal the exact nature of the problem concerning TS's gregariousness, or what failures in professionalism have been shown. The central complaint is not adequately described, and it is unclear why TS has been referred at all, given that the matter was originally dealt with locally.

At the interview stage, the committee has to rely largely on TS's account, and while questions remain as to why he was referred in the first place, it is generally appropriate that no further action is going to be taken. What happened with the letter in the hospital is bad enough, and the committee does not want to compound the difficulties currently being faced by TS.

The substantive issue concerning unacceptable behaviours in the operating room was never made clear and, perhaps wisely, TS chose to remain silent on this point. Given a considerable power imbalance that exists, there is more than a suspicion that TS is being 'hung out to dry' in order to protect the surgeon. Additionally, there is the possible inequity between the way in which the other two students are being dealt with as compared with TS, in that they were never referred on to the committee. Also unresolved is the question of why TS's apparent gregariousness is such as issue. The head of the clinical programme's explanation about the surgeon's behaviour, making reference to the natural 'pecking order', leaves one wondering what the agenda is with regard to a situation, the dynamics of which include the possibility that TS is a target for restless energy that has been accumulating in the wake of recent 'events'.

The hospital director seemed to overreact in telling TS that his behaviour was unacceptable, adding that his future in medicine was at risk in the event of further misbehaviour, which is a strong statement, given what has been said about other members of staff. TS has been exposed to a number of negative role models, and the hospital director victimised him without really knowing the facts. Furthermore, the head of the clinical programme failed to intervene to ensure equity between all the students who were present in the operating room. If the nurses' complaint is to be taken at face value, then nobody stood up to defend TS against unreasonable and inequitable action.

While the PCC rightly considered that further action was unnecessary and unlikely to produce any benefit (possibly only leading to even further intimidation of TS), the question remains as to whether something further could have been done for TS, and whether the behaviour of the head of the clinical programme and the hospital director should have been more robustly challenged. The nurses' action in complaining about the students but not the doctor is probably reflective of a hierarchical culture that tends to protect those at the top while damaging those nearer 'the bottom of the pile'. Above all, taking appropriate action should help to ensure that humiliated students do not learn to behave like their role models, in so doing perpetuating an unprofessional culture.

In addition to the negative aspects of role modelling and the toxicity of traditional hierarchical professional culture, the case illustrates the importance of clear communication and the necessity of taking into account the *context* of behaviours when trying to assess their *nature*.[5,6] Without attention to these factors, students can be at a distinct disadvantage, and medical schools should be mindful of this possibility and ensure that student professionalism processes do not reinforce the unethical behaviours that they are attempting to prevent. Instead, schools should protect students from victimisation and contribute to the lifelong learning of qualified staff and the clinical educators who should have known better. Failures in professionalism can be found at all levels and are not limited to trainees. Implied racist elements of the original conversation were never disclosed, and TS was at risk of being made a scapegoat for other people's unacceptable behaviours.

Summary

- Students are subject to influence by role models at every turn. Failure to subject staff to the same processes as students demonstrates double standards, entrenching the more corrosive aspects of medical culture.
- Students are at risk of being victimised for behaviour that may have complex causes. It is important to understand the full context of unprofessional behaviour among students; without this process, the outcome of a case such as this seems unfair.
- There is no evidence of patient safety being an issue in this case.
- Communication, including referrals of student professionalism issues, should be concise and comprehensive, and any complaint has to be justified. While it is difficult to be objective when assessing complaints, all relevant parties should be invited to present their views.
- Medical schools owe students protection from victimisation by senior staff, and where such behaviour is found, schools should expose and reject it in order to avoid the risk of perpetuating the unjust hierarchical aspects of medical culture.
- Regulators are no doubt aware that such issues arise from time to time; however, it does not become their province unless or until the local avenues have been exhausted. Complaints that have a public interest component merit proper investigation.
- Guidelines were not an issue in this case.

CASE 26

A medical student has doubtful long-term goals and an objection to vaccinations.

Outline

A first-year medical student, YM, fails to submit evidence that she has achieved immune status to a range of infectious diseases, including diphtheria, pertussis, hepatitis B, measles, mumps and rubella. Local health providers require all health professional staff to be immune to such infections as a condition of entering their facilities and having contact with patients. This requirement is a clause in the contract for student clinical placements, some of which take place for YM in the upcoming semester. Unlike some students in this situation, who might be just a little disorganised, YM tells the administration office that she is unable to comply because she and her family are conscientious objectors to vaccinations on the grounds of belief – namely, that vaccinations can be harmful to health. As a compromise, YM offers to try a homoeopathic hepatitis B vaccination under her father's guidance; this involves drinking a solution of extremely dilute (but increasingly concentrated) live hepatitis virus over a period of 6 months. An infectious diseases physician is consulted, and he rejects this approach as being non-evidence based, and the student is referred to the year convener to discuss the situation.

YM's father is a homoeopath and he sends with her copies of research papers from a homoeopathy journal, allegedly proving the danger of vaccinations. Furthermore, YM states that a cousin had an unusual neurological illness as a child that the family blames on his vaccinations and furnishes a supporting letter from the treating neurologist. However, this letter is a photocopy of a photocopy of a document dated 10 years ago stating that the illness was unexplained. YM is reminded that this requirement was part of an information pack sent out to all applicants upon receiving an offer of placement at the medical school; the position is clearly stated on the medical school website, and the policy conforms to national medical education standards. YM responds by saying that she is only studying medicine so that she can later practise as a homoeopath. She simply wants the professional recognition and is not a believer in allopathic medicine. YM still declines to comply, and she is referred to the school's Health and Professional Conduct Committee (HPCC). Prior to the HPCC meeting, the family contacts the university with a threat of legal action on grounds of discrimination if she is forced to have the 'approved' vaccinations.

At the HPCC she restates her case, but the committee confirms the school's decision that this requirement *must* be met, and that she will be unable to progress further without doing her clinical placements, which require vaccination. Realising she has hit a barrier, YM asks for time to reflect on the issue. She is unsure how to proceed, and in order to try to put pressure on the medical school she starts an online discussion group complaining of bias and discriminatory attitudes towards alternative and complementary medicine. She carefully reads the websites of other medical schools in the state and finds one where the wording regarding vaccination is a little more open. Meanwhile, her father obtains legal advice and is told that he would be unlikely to win a case if it went to court.

The year convener calls YM in for a further meeting, pressing her for a decision, and YM asks for reassurance that if she has the vaccinations she will not be treated unfairly by the staff. The school agrees to take no further action so long as she complies. However, her father has told her that he will not continue to financially support her if she fails to respect family values and beliefs and that she will have to fund herself through the rest of the programme. Amid these pressures she applies for leave from the programme, and a year later she recommences a medical course at another university.

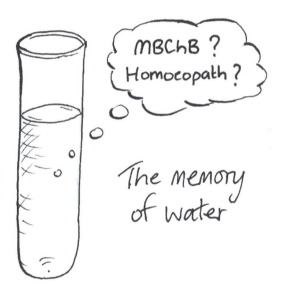

Questions

- What are the arguments for health professional students having immunity to such infectious diseases?
- How strong is the evidence on homoeopathic vaccination, and what (if anything) do medical schools need to consider? Should the school have acted differently?
- How do we balance individual rights against population rights on an issue such as this?

Discussion

While this case includes issues such as family dynamics, it is really about rights and responsibilities. Medical curricula are required to inform medical students about complementary and alternative medicine (CAM), even if only as part of an approach to ensure that medical graduates practise evidence-based medicine, regardless of its origin.* Curriculum standards include wording such as 'based upon principles of scientific method and evidence-based practice', and fostering 'analytical and critical thinking'. This recognises the evidence that exists about safety and efficacy and contemporary management strategies where there is little or no record of patient harm.[7]

However, CAM is popular with patients, and individual practitioners have the right to their own beliefs, so long as standards of practice are considered safe and appropriate. It could be acceptable for an individual medical student (or medical practitioner) to accept the personal risk of being exposed, without immunity, to infectious diseases among their patients. On the other hand, public health considerations must be taken into account. First, there is the potential for non-immune health professionals to transmit infectious diseases in the workplace, and so non-vaccinated healthcare workers pose a risk to patient safety. Employers and health sector managers are increasingly reluctant to accept such risks, and health professionals have to be aware of this. Second, 'herd immunity' (or critical mass within the community as a whole) is more difficult to achieve if health professionals do not act as role models and advocate compliance with recommended vaccination schedules. The consequence of students being able to follow their own route and only have vaccinations that they 'believe in' would be unworkable from both a legal and a public health perspective. As a result, there are requirements for medical schools to have clear policies on managing infectious disease risks. Increasingly, requirements of these policies are included in codes of conduct or agreements that entrants into medical school must sign.

The school takes a strong stand because it has no other option; there is a signed contract with local health providers that would expose the school to legal action if a student became involved in a disease outbreak. No working arrangement with local health providers means no clinical placements, or, to put it another way, no working arrangement with local health providers means no school of medicine; no vaccinations means no medical students on the wards and hence no clinical practice experience.

In this case utility and the rights of the community as a whole must trump individual freedoms of expression. However, YM was not disciplined for starting a more open discussion about the topic. While the school applied a certain

---

* The Australian Medical Council released new guidance on this in early 2013 as part of a revision of standards for undergraduate medical education.

degree of pressure, it was family pressure that eventually led to her withdrawal, and in this respect there was no way that the school could intervene.[8]

Summary

- While complementary and alternative medicine approaches are popular with patients and with some practitioners, the school has contractual and moral obligations to insist on YM being vaccinated. Her unprofessionalism arose from failing to comply with a policy to which she had signed up, not because of her beliefs.
- The outcome was neither intended nor desirable, but it was probably unavoidable given the circumstances.
- Patient safety and public protection are central to this case; the school has a legal and a moral duty to require students to comply.
- This case is not about education and training other than to the extent that it challenges attitudes and beliefs towards other, less conventional forms of medicine.
- Systems to ensure students comply with required immunisations and protocols seemed to work well in this case.
- The case raises issues about public health and policy, and these were dealt with effectively at local level.
- Students have a duty to protect members of the public from infectious diseases; professional guidelines require this type of compliance.

CASE 27

A member of the public says a medical student is using drugs and collecting guns.

Outline

AD, a 21-year-old medical student, comes to the attention of the school midway through the course. His progress has been reasonable to date and no specific concerns have been noted. However, a member of the public who knows this student telephones the school, saying that she is concerned about his recreational use of marijuana, and the fact that he collects guns. The informant does not want to put any of her concerns in writing but she is happy for her name to be used when talking with the student. A senior administrator speaks with the student, and his version of events is that he enjoys recreational hunting and has a legal gun licence. On the other issue, he eventually admits to using marijuana, and he agrees to see a psychiatrist specialising in addictions and for a report to be sent to the medical school.

A psychiatric review does not uncover any major issues regarding drug abuse; however, it is noted that the student shows high levels of social anxiety. At the same time, a number of course conveners are reporting frequent absences from clinical placements, and ultimately he fails the year. When interviewed, he reveals that he is anxious and guarded around fellow students and with patients and that he is ambivalent about pursuing medicine as a career. He decides to take a year out from medical school, and in the end he does not return.

Questions

- How should a school respond to complaints against a medical student brought by a concerned member of the public?
- How can medical schools identify and deal with students who lack the motivation needed to pursue a career in medicine?
- Is it wrong for a medical student or trainee to own guns, and how important is drug use to the case?

Discussion

That a member of the public raised the initial concern illustrates a difficult dilemma with regard to where a medical school's jurisdiction begins and ends. Clearly, unprofessional behaviours that occur within a medical school setting fall within the medical school's purview. Similarly, the school should know about (and act upon) unprofessional behaviours that occur outside a medical school setting and that affect medical school performance. The difficulty here is that the school has to be careful not to interfere in a student's private life, and it can only make a judgement *after* gathering sufficient information, which of necessity means asking questions about the student's private life. If the student had collected guns illegally and had unlawful intent, the school would undoubtedly need to know, just as if a student is trading in illegal drugs and/or his performance is affected by the use of drugs, the school needs to know. The difficulty for any school is in 'knowing when it needs to know'.

The Medical Council of New Zealand (MCNZ) states that illegal use of drugs by doctors is a matter that should be brought to its attention; even though use of recreational marijuana in New Zealand is illegal, the law is not strongly enforced for the general public. While abuse of prescription drugs is not infrequently brought to the attention of the MCNZ, use of recreational drugs rarely gives rise to a major complaint or investigation. Thus, there is a grey zone between what is regarded as unlawful and what is regarded as socially unacceptable and/or unethical. Gathering relevant information is crucial, and such investigations can only be undertaken once a medical school believes that a threshold requiring it to act has been crossed. This leads to a double bind – to investigate and ignore privacy, or to do nothing and ignore concerns that have been raised. From the public's perspective, the latter is not a viable option, and if something went seriously wrong it could lead to civil and possibly criminal charges relating to the school's public and professional responsibilities.

A medical student or trainee might well ask, 'am I ever off duty?' The answer is that it depends on the nature and gravity of the concerns. For example, if it turned out that the guns had not been legal, then not only does the medical school need to know but also the school would have to inform the police. However, a possibility exists that complaints made by members of the public are vexatious, and in that case, making strenuous enquiries and invading the student's privacy could be seen as unnecessarily intrusive.

In the present case, the medical school decided to meet with the student, who understood the dilemmas faced by the medical school and was surprisingly open when the complaint was first discussed. Given his deteriorating performance following this conversation, and his cautious, anxious demeanour when talking with the administration, many unanswered questions remain. While the complaint was taken at face value, in retrospect it most likely represents underlying problems that had previously not been identified, including ambivalence about pursuing a career in medicine and a possible social phobia. Whether the problems would have been remediable had they come to light earlier is not known. Absence from the course is often a marker of other problems, and schools need to be alert to this possibility. In this case, calling the student in earlier in order to assess what was behind the absences would have been the best course of action.

Summary

- The boundary between a student's private life and medical school life is not always clear; in terms of professionalism, the distinction may not matter since both areas are relevant.
- Inquiring into a student's private life may be seen as intrusive; while fairness requires the right to privacy to be respected, the interests of justice require public interest to be considered, thus overriding the right to privacy.
- When a member of the public raises concerns it can be difficult to determine the appropriate level of inquiry; however, patient safety cannot be ignored. Schools should proceed with caution but should not ignore the complaint.
- Unexplained absences from educational and training exercises are often a marker for other problems; this should be borne in mind and monitored, where appropriate.
- Protocol is important, and procedures may need checking to ensure that public interest and rights to privacy are balanced against each other in relation to possible risks.

- The regulator needs to be told about relevant information that could be used later in an investigation, especially if there are public interest concerns.
- Inconsistencies between legal and ethical standards regarding recreational drug use are part of the problem in this case; as a matter of public policy the issue may need revisiting.

CASE 28

A medical student is rather keen to gain experience on an international elective.

Outline

At the end of his penultimate year of study, ME, a medical student, travels to a developing nation for an elective clinical placement, comprising 8 weeks of clinical experience under the supervision of a local medical practitioner. He negotiated this placement via a local charity that has connections with a rural hospital, which has relatively few professional staff. He stayed on afterwards for an adventure holiday, and on returning to Australia he boasts to his friends about the amazing opportunities he had and the confidence that he gained. He claims that he 'ran the hospital alone over one weekend when the supervising clinicians were exhausted and needed a break'. He had to make decisions about when to perform procedures, such as general anaesthesia, fracture setting and instrumental obstetrics, and he even performed a caesarean section with help from the nurses.

His elective placement supervisor report is reasonably positive about his work ethic and commitment, but it includes a vague statement suggesting that he was not good at recognising his limits; this comment is reflective of patient complications that occurred due to his poorly supervised actions. There is also a comment about the student's tendency to get overinvolved in local health politics; for example, he led complaints at a local community meeting about the poor workforce situation and the resulting poor healthcare. The electives convener is worried about these comments and calls the student in to discuss them. The student is dismissive of the concerns, stating that the patients received care that was 'better than none at all' and that the nurses and orderlies were very good. He goes on to say that the requirements of the elective placement programme are vague and that many students attended much less diligently than he did. Nonetheless, as a result of his apparently poor insight, ME is referred to the Health and Professional Conduct Committee (HPCC), which finds by a narrow margin that his behaviour was unprofessional; it concludes by saying that the student must complete a further 8-week elective placement in more controlled conditions prior to graduation. This decision will not only delay his graduation but also cause financial loss, both because he will have to fund another trip and because it will delay the start of paid work as a trainee doctor.

ME appeals the decision at the University Appeals Committee, which overturns the decision on the grounds that the requirements of clinical electives are so vague that there is insufficient evidence to support a fail decision.

Questions
- What supervision is expected for elective clinical placements in a developing nation, and how does this differ from placements in well-resourced nations?
- What are the risks for this student if a serious adverse outcome arises from a case that he was involved in while on placement?
- To what extent is it appropriate for a student to become involved in local health politics?
- What does the story suggest about ME's attitude towards professionalism?
- Does the initial decision of the HPCC seem fair and proportionate, and is it fair that ME takes all the blame?

Discussion

This case raises issues for the individual concerned in terms of professionalism, but it also raises wider issues having to do with standards and policy for international electives. While here is not the place to debate the issues in full, the problems encountered by this student are not unique and do need to be addressed. Educators with involvement in organising placements will no doubt have encountered similar difficulties, and lack of clarity on how best to approach the problem is serious and warranting of attention.[9]

Medical students often travel to countries with less-developed systems of healthcare than the ones with which they are familiar; it is quite likely that students will find themselves in a situation whereby they do not want to refuse anyone care but neither do they want to overstep their bounds and land themselves in trouble. In addition, the opportunity to gain experience is attractive and potentially fulfilling. In this case, the student went a step further and tried to organise some action to improve care at the local level. This was no doubt well motivated, but possibly unwise, given that his commitment was necessarily short-lived and his lack of knowledge about factors influencing how the local health economy and society works.

While there is an element of universality about ethical standards, at a practical level there is often a gulf between what codes of practice theoretically demand and the standards expected and upheld by local healthcare providers. On one hand, you could argue that there is only one thing more dangerous than a doctor or trainee who does not know what he is doing (the *consciously incompetent*), and that is a doctor who thinks he knows what he is doing but in reality does not (the *unconsciously incompetent*). On the other hand, there is validity to the point, implied by ME, that without him patients could otherwise go without care or experience unreasonably long delays. Is care provided by someone inexperienced better or worse than having no care at all? While this question does not have an answer, we need to think about professional standards and expectations in this kind of setting and consider the question of jurisdiction.

While the local care facility will primarily be responsible for standards of patient care and safety and for defending itself in terms of clinical negligence, the student is representing his school, and it has no bearing on whether he is providing care in a hospital in his home town or in a remote rural village. In addition, if levels of local healthcare provision are poor, it is possibly also the case that access to justice may be inadequate; while that may be true, the question that concerns us here is not about negligence or access to justice but *professionalism* and lack of judgement in working beyond one's competence. Guidelines clearly state that doctors (and by implication medical students) must work within the limits of their competence, and while geography should not make any difference to how those standards are applied, practical realities make a difference to how things work on the ground.[7]

Context and social setting do make a difference in terms of how care is provided, by whom and to what standard, and students should recognise this. They also need to recognise that when they are on a placement, their home school has a devolved responsibility for both their behaviour and the local care that they help provide. ME was perhaps overenthusiastic and lacked insight into the appropriateness of his actions, and it is right that he is asked to explain. However, if there is lack of clarity as to what standards apply in remote settings and how to respond to demands from patients and from other providers of care, then the student is not the one who is at fault. In general, there is no consistency on this point in terms of clarity and sensibility of standards and expectations.

In this particular case, the HPCC probably took a harsh view. It was right and fully within its powers to draw attention to ME's lack of professionalism, but to cause him to delay graduation with the consequences that followed would seem to be putting blame on his shoulders without properly acknowledging a much wider problem. The decision of the Appeals Committee was in some ways unfortunate but probably understandable, as well as fair, given that overseas clinical electives are relatively unregulated.

In the current legal climate, it would be wise for medical schools to develop more precise supervision, scope of practice and assessment guidelines for these placements. In order to defend appeals, these guidelines should be consistent with those of other clinical placements and with regulations of the broader university environment; in our view, the era of relatively unregulated international electives may be drawing to a close. Schools must carefully balance the need for a 'coming of age' experience with requirements for graduated supervision and workplace-based assessment.

Summary

- Professionalism in context and the extent to which standards can and should be applied in different settings are central to this case.
- On the available evidence, ME suffered from insufficiently clear guidance being in place for dealing with issues of this kind.
- Patient safety and public protection always matter, even in remote settings; but how standards are upheld could well be influenced by what is realistically achievable.
- Educators need to be aware of situations to which students find themselves exposed; giving students clear guidance before they set off doing international electives must surely be considered.
- Protocol matters, and while it was generally fit for purpose in this case, the fact that the case was overturned on appeal indicates a mismatch between standards expected by the central university and those set by the school.
- There is some awareness that public bodies need to tackle the underlying issues arising from this case, and it is an area that merits further work.
- We have no information about local guidelines, but it was not clear to students how far standards learned in class should apply in settings that differ substantially from those to which they are accustomed.

CASE 29

A junior medical student with prior experience wants to do more advanced work.

Outline

DP is a 34-year-old international medical student in his first year at a graduate-entry medical school; he has previous work experience as a paramedic. He opts to travel to a South East Asian country for a 4-week elective with four other students. The hospital director in the provincial town they selected meets the students and asks about what areas they would like to work in. DP chooses to start in paediatric outpatients, which is supervised by a nurse practitioner (NP). He is given a desk and the NP announces, 'Here's your first patient'. DP soon discovers that he is expected to write prescriptions for the hospital pharmacy and order investigations.

He expresses concern about this situation to his colleagues, who, after all, are only first-year medical students. However, he enjoys the hands-on experience, as that is one of the features that helped him decide on a Third World country for his elective. His paramedic experience combined with having spent years in the military, as well as having 'advice' from the NP, makes him feel reasonably confident. After 2 weeks he moves on to the adult emergency department, which is supposed to be supervised by a doctor, but it turns out that the supervisor is a third-year medical student from the United Kingdom.

DP finds the hospital extremely run-down and with very poor medical equipment; it is short on staffing and supplies and it is run by a seemingly dysfunctional government health department, with a hospital director who is mostly preoccupied by lobbying for medical supplies. While the students had been told that there would be regular educational activities during their stay, this does not occur. At the end of the elective the NP, the third-year medical student and a surgeon who observed DP during the final part of the elective sign DP's attendance forms. Finally, the hospital director completes the student evaluation report, but it is based on the advice of the other staff, since the surgeon in charge is rarely in the hospital.

On his arrival home, DP receives a letter from the medical school requiring him to attend an interview with the Professional Conduct Committee. Two of his student colleagues have written to the school, indicating their concerns that DP saw a number of patients without supervision and appeared to be diagnosing patients, as well as ordering investigations and writing prescriptions. The students indicated that DP continued doing this *after* they had spoken to him about the matter. They said that DP did not seem concerned that this was potentially harmful to patients, pointing out that it could be a bad learning experience for *him*. They explained how the hospital failed to understand what 'being a first-year student' meant in terms of how little students really knew.

At interview, DP asserts that he never exceeded his abilities as a first-year student, and that the NP was always present in outpatients. He assures the committee that he never caused harm to patients, and that the hospital director, when asked, assured him that he was doing fine. He adds that members of the hospital staff were grateful to him for his contribution, congratulating him on being professional, hard-working and knowledgeable. Therefore, DP finds it astounding and unacceptable that student peers have 'whistle-blown' him to the school, especially when they were attached to different departments within the hospital. After interviewing DP, the committee informs him that he is required to hold regular meetings with a mentor during his second year, in order to review and monitor his professionalism; furthermore, during any forthcoming elective periods tutors will be asked to provide close supervision.

Questions

- Who is most to blame in this situation?
- Is it acceptable to countenance differing standards of professionalism in different settings?
- How feasible is it to monitor and audit international placements, especially if they are arranged directly by the student?

Discussion

Medical students increasingly travel overseas for international healthcare experiences; this is part of a trend towards developing breadth in medical training. It also helps to attract international students to the school and to equip graduates to work anywhere in the world. Schools offer a variety of elective placements, and they encourage experiences that provide contrasting experiences from their First World programmes, with the opportunity to experience new and interesting places. This much is positive, but DP is one of many students who encounter a situation that is increasingly recognised as posing risks to patients, students and schools. Clinical training is being brought forward into the hitherto 'preclinical' years, with the result that clinical electives increasingly involve students in the early stages of their training.[10]

The maturity of DP possibly gave him added credibility in the eyes of local professional staff; in addition, the elective hospital was apparently poorly resourced. In combination, the fact that the director was often not present and provided no direct teaching or supervision but was still prepared to sign off student evaluations raises questions about whether or not this was a suitable placement, especially for such an inexperienced student. In elective situations that have poorly resourced facilities, it could be argued that local staff are taking advantage of students from developed countries simply because they are prepared to work in these very challenging situations.[11,12]

Students in these situations are vulnerable, partly because as students they are at the bottom of the pack in the hierarchy of medical practice, and partly because they are relatively young and very inexperienced. Keenness to gain experience can make students less vigilant about remaining within the boundaries of acceptable practice. Patient safety was never seriously considered, and it seems that at the local level, the prevailing view is that receiving treatment from a medical student is better than receiving no treatment at all.

However, this may not be the case, and it does not absolve medical students from their professional responsibility or accountability towards their teachers back home. Furthermore, medical schools themselves are not without responsibility for allowing students to go on placements that are poorly supervised and resourced. One could argue, therefore, that the moral blame is split three ways among student, school and local provider; however, on this occasion, the only person in trouble is a student in his first year at medical school.

Issues of objectivity arose in two main areas. First, perfunctory sign-off by hospital staff who failed to provide proper feedback to students about their performance. Second, having students take responsibility for patient care with uncertain levels of supervision put patients at risk of potential harm. DP's self-confidence notwithstanding, the risk of exceeding his abilities and causing harm to patients is very real, and he appears to suffer from the well-known syndrome of 'not knowing what you don't know'. This is compounded by assurances received from the hospital director and other clinical staff. Overall, this bodes ill for DP's capacity to recognise when he needs to ask for help, a requirement that is an important skill in modern medical practice.[13,14] It also bodes ill for the medical school and for any future students going to this location, to say nothing of patients themselves.

Unbeknown to them, students could be being placed in a dangerous medico-legal situation, in the event that they provide care that results in patient harm. While students are usually protected by the home university's insurance, there is a degree of complexity and uncertainty in this area in terms of who is covered and for what eventuality. The fact that there have been very few incidents so far is no cause for complacency. Schools should be explicit about where the boundaries of liability lie, and they owe it to partner institutions and to their students to carry out some form of placement audit before students are assigned. Overall, it is likely that this process falls well short of what is necessary, especially given the speed at which overseas student electives are currently increasing in popularity.[15]

This case combines the problem of an apparently overconfident student, which must be determined by careful and sympathetic discussion at interview, with that of common risks attending an overseas student placement. Risks of patient and student harm are multiplied when an overconfident student works in a setting that is not adequately staffed, prepared or supervised. Placements such as this may take advantage of student vulnerability, particularly when someone is overconfident, and when they are used to supplement local staffing inadequacies. Students might see this as an opportunity, but they need sufficient insight to know that they remain professionally accountable. While the school is not without blame, it may provide a lesson for DP to have moderate sanctions imposed by the committee.

Summary

- Medical students often spend elective time in international healthcare settings; this increasingly happens during the early years of training, and neither the school nor the student seemed aware of the accompanying hazards until professionalism issues were highlighted by the other students.

- Elective host institutions may be poorly resourced, with uneven clinical supervision for students. Schools should take a more active part in where students go on international (and, to some extent, national) electives, and local staff need to be suitably trained and at hand.

- Patient safety and public protection matter in every setting, but if local healthcare providers have limited regard for these issues or are unaware of limits to students' knowledge and experience, this is an issue in itself. Students have to learn how best to respond and should receive preparation prior to embarking on such an elective.

- Poor educational experiences, inappropriate levels of responsibility and medico-legal risks are problems that could face any student on a clinical elective. Some settings are more hazardous than others, and the home institution needs to be aware of these difficulties.

- Adequate pre-placement preparation and instruction are crucial; it is the school's responsibility to ensure that the placement satisfies minimum educational and safety standards. Procedures need to be in place for auditing placements wherever they occur.

- While such matters are for individual schools to address, regulators can also play a role in encouraging schools to be vigilant.

- No international guidelines are applicable to these situations, other than those set by bodies such as the World Medical Association.[16]

REFERENCES

1. Gabbard GO, Nadelson C. Professional boundaries in the physician-patient relationship. *JAMA*. 1995; **273**(18): 1445–9.
2. Australian Higher Education Occupational Physicians / Practitioners Society. *Medical Students: standards of medical fitness to train*. HEOPS; 2011. Available at: www.heops. org.uk/HEOPS_Medical_Students_fitness_standards_2011_v7.pdf (accessed 10 June 2013).
3. General Medical Council. Relationships with patients. *Medical Students: professional values and fitness to practise*. London: GMC; 2009. §§ 23–28. Available at: www.gmc-uk.org/education/undergraduate/professional_behaviour.asp (accessed 17 February 2013).
4. General Medical Council. Working with colleagues. *Medical Students: professional values and fitness to practise*. London: GMC; 2009. §§ 29–32. Available at: www.gmc-uk.org/education/undergraduate/professional_behaviour.asp (accessed 17 February 2013).
5. Rees CE, Knight LV. The trouble with assessing students' professionalism: theoretical insights from sociocognitive psychology. *Acad Med*. 2007; **82**(1): 46–50.
6. Rees CE, Knight LV. Banning, detection, attribution and reaction: the role of asses-

sors in constructing students' unprofessional behaviours. *Med Educ.* 2008; **42**(2): 125–7.

7. Australian Medical Council. *Accreditation Standards for Primary Medical Education Providers and their Program of Study and Graduate Outcome Statements.* Kingston, ACT: AMC [updated 17 January 2013]. Available at: www.amc.org.au/images/ Accreditation/FINAL-Standards-and-Graduate-Outcome-Statements-20-December-2012.pdf (accessed 10 June 2013).

8. Australian Medical Council. *Graduate Outcome Statement: professionalism and leadership.* Kingston, ACT: AMC. Available at: www.amc.org.au/ (accessed 17 February 2013).

9. Anderson KC, Slatnik MA, Pereira I, *et al.* Are we there yet? Preparing Canadian students for global health electives. *Acad Med.* 2012; **87**(2): 206–9.

10. Jake Parker, Rob Mitchell, Sarah Mansfield, *et al.* Launch of 'A guide to working abroad for Australian medical students and junior doctors'. *Med J Aust.* 2011; **195**(1): 44. Available at: www.mja.com.au/journal/2011/195/1/launch-guide-working-abroad-australian-medical-students-and-junior-doctors (accessed 17 February 2013).

11. Elit L, Hunt M, Redwood-Campbell L, *et al.* Ethical issues encountered by medical students during international health electives. *Med Educ.* 2011; **45**(7): 704–11.

12. Petrosoniak A, McCarthy A, Varpio L. International health electives: thematic results of student and professional interviews. *Med Educ.* 2010; **44**(7): 683–9.

13. General Medical Council. *Tomorrow's Doctors: outcomes 3; the doctor as a professional.* London: GMC; 2009. Available at: www.gmc-uk.org/education/undergraduate/ tomorrows_doctors_2009_outcomes3.asp (accessed 17 February 2013).

14. Australian Medical Council. *Accreditation Standards for Medical Schools and their Programs of Study: attributes of medical graduates.* Kingston, ACT: AMC; 2013. §33. Available at: www.amc.org.au/images/Medschool/accreditation-standards-medical-schools-2010.pdf (accessed 17 February 2013).

15. Murdoch-Eaton D, Green A. The contribution and challenges of electives in the development of social accountability in medical students. *Med Teach.* 2011; **33**(8): 643–8.

16. World Medical Association. *WMA International Code of Medical Ethics.* Geneva: WMA; 2006. Available at: www.wma.net/en/30publications/10policies/c8/ (accessed 17 February 2013).

CHAPTER 8

Postscript

Reflections on the cases as a whole, including comments on current trends and suggestions for best practice for developing policies and procedures.

REFLECTIONS ON THE CASES

The full collection of cases provides an overview of some of the main issues featuring in cases that come before professionalism committees and disciplinary panels. Recognising that cases have been fictionalised as well as anonymised and that stories behind the various narratives happened over time, they are based on reality and some issues feature with relative frequency (e.g. drug-related and mental health problems, as well as general issues relating to poor performance).

When inviting case contributions, we did not stipulate the topics that we wanted covered. If some topics occur more than others it is perhaps either because professionalism committees address them more often or because they present in a more complex way and so are harder to resolve. We thought of filtering out cases to prevent duplication, but this would have distorted the 'truth' in terms of what is going on. However, there is no attempt to present the cases as 'evidence', and they are not the product of any form of systematic research.

One issue that we possibly underplay in terms of the topics covered concerns the use of social networking sites. Committees around the world are in the process of working out how best to respond to problems relating to inappropriate postings online, and guidance regarding how best to deal with professionalism issues associated with this phenomenon is only just being developed. This emphasises the fact that schools and programmes need to ensure that their procedures and protocols are generally up to date and fit for purpose.

Problems associated with the application of new technology rarely become apparent straight away; there is invariably a time delay after their introduction. Besides, our contributors are not writing about cases that are coming up now; they are reflecting on cases that came up in the recent past. Additionally, the law tends to be slow in responding to challenges about what is or is not permissible, and ethical frameworks also take time to be developed and updated. Therefore, educators need to find effective ways of dealing with new problems as and when they arise.

A point worth noting, which only became visible after the cases were written, is that the caseload in US schools and programmes appears to be smaller than in the United Kingdom, Australia or New Zealand. Once again, there is no attempt to present this as 'fact', and it may just be coincidence; however, it appears that in the United States, more day-to-day professionalism issues are dealt with as and when they occur, without requiring a trainee to have to appear before a panel of inquiry. The North American cases are all relatively complex, and they present with issues that took place over time. When a hearing is convened it probably means that the matter has already been discussed 'in context', and that only when it is sufficiently serious as to require escalation does it come to a committee's attention. Again, this perception is based on our observations, nothing more.

Another point worth noting is that all applicants to medical school in the United States have been through a minimum of 4 years of undergraduate higher education. This means that they have slightly greater maturity than their counterparts in the other countries, where graduate entry to medical school only accounts for a minority of applicants. Under that system, a junior doctor will be entering postgraduate education at the age of 23 or 24 as opposed to 27 or 28, which clearly makes a difference in terms of life experience.

Finally, it is becoming clear that students and trainees increasingly bring in lawyers to challenge disciplinary decisions made by committees. While this used to be a rare occurrence, that is no longer the case. Legal involvement is not to be feared, and it can help promote fairness and prevent unreasonable or biased decisions from being made, as well as helping to prevent unnecessary appeals. However, it can have the effect of protracting a case and increasing costs (emotionally and materially).

The best way that a school or programme can protect itself is to take appropriate steps to ensure that its systems and procedures are legally compliant, up to date and, of course, adhered to. If a school does not have appropriate procedures in place, or if it does not follow them when they do exist, it is asking for decisions to be overturned. It is not that we are siding with programme directors or committee chairs as a matter of policy; it is rather that when a case is overturned on a technicality it can potentially lead to an unprofessional and/or unsafe person being allowed to progress and go on to practise medicine. This makes for neither good educational practice nor sound public policy.

DEVELOPING PROCESSES AND PROCEDURES TO GUIDE THE DEVELOPMENT OF SOUND PROFESSIONALISM IN LEARNERS

Unprofessionalism can harm patients and have an adverse effect on teams. The real challenge is finding effective, appropriate and workable ways of teaching and assessing professionalism. This can be done concurrently with ensuring the provision of suitable role models so that the next generation of clinicians is equipped to take its place in society. A feature of the range of cases presented in this book is that they are all difficult to manage, regardless of location, level of education or scope of clinical experience. The relationships between initial presentations, underlying issues and outcomes are subtle and complex, and using diagrammatic form, Table 8.1 illustrates how some of these relations work.

After investigation, most presentations of poor professionalism can be caused by one or more underlying issues. Then, depending on processes for balancing various rights and responsibilities and the options that are available in managing a problem, eventual outcomes could vary considerably. The steps of investigation and later judgement are important parts of the process for managing potential breaches of professionalism. Based on our own experience in health professional education and regulation, the following 10 steps can be used as a guide to managing professionalism within medical education institutions.

1. *Ground the regulations in current professional codes of conduct.* Policy incoherence is bad for students and trainees as well as for programmes and schools. If heads of school or programme directors adopt appropriate guidelines, consistent with current thinking and best practice, it is less likely that they will be challenged, and it helps in promoting a general culture of fairness.

2. *Engage with patient groups and students to incorporate their perspectives and gain their support for implementation.* An inclusive approach to policy-setting makes good sense and can result in better policy and guidance by reflecting the interests of all the different parties concerned. That is, patients and public need to be involved as well as students and trainees.

3. *Panels that make decisions need to be broadly based and include representatives of the wider community and peers of the learners being assessed.* Panel or committee members might need professional development training, but this does not mean that membership should be restricted to senior members of staff. As with policy-setting, the process should be open and socially inclusive.

TABLE 8.1 Presentations, underlying issues and outcomes: complex relationships

Presenting complaint		Underlying issue		Outcome
Unexplained absences	*Investigation to gain greater understanding*	Poor motivation	*Judgement about management options*	No formal measures
Persistent lateness		Dishonesty		Proceed with specific remediation
Poor organisational skills		Alcohol misuse		Time out for reflection
Poor clinical performance		Other drug misuse		Specific treatment options
Poor teamwork		Attention deficit hyperactivity disorder		Suspension
Criminal procedures		Autism spectrum disorder		Expulsion
		Personality disorder		
		Depression		
		Bipolar		
		Psychosis		

There needs to be continuity of process, starting with policy-setting and following through to implementation and appeal, where appropriate.

4. *Align regulations and processes for managing breaches in health professional schools carefully with those of the whole educational institution and/or healthcare organisation.* There should be internal consistency and alignment in terms of protocols operating within a university and within local healthcare provider institutions; this is not easy to achieve, since the goals of a university and the goals of a teaching hospital are not the same. Meaningful dialogue and exchange of information should help to bridge this gap.

5. *Seek legal advice to achieve the correct wording that minimises misinterpretation; regulations have to be strong enough to withstand appeals based on discrimination against disability, health, gender, ethnicity, religion and age.* This additional step might incur upfront cost, but it pays off later on if legal challenges are mounted against decisions made by investigating committees. Furthermore, committees should be open to the possibility of legal challenges being made on the basis of alleged human rights violations.

6. *Encourage learners to seek independent legal advice in proceedings against them. While protecting their interests, timely legal advice should help dispel possible false hopes of winning an appeal.* If regulations and processes are clear, open and followed, independent legal advice rarely identifies legitimate grounds for lodging an appeal. Appeals are founded on errors of process rather than on re-examination of the facts; being aware of this can help learners to accept decisions when they are made.

7. *Carefully consider which circumstances can be accepted as counting towards mitigation. Without guidance and appropriate evidence, mitigation can become a source of 'gaming' by appellants and their representatives.* Ideally, advise staff and trainees about timelines (i.e. up to and until which time mitigating circumstances can be accepted). Being clear and transparent helps everyone involved in the business of judging cases and hearing appeals. Mitigating circumstances are sometimes valid and entirely plausible; schools and programmes need to apply the rules with fairness and discretion.

8. *Where possible, encourage and reward honesty by learners who have made mistakes – although a reward should only include 'absolution' in less serious cases.* Just like anyone else, doctors in training are going to make mistakes; something that potentially differentiates professionals from other people is having the ability to recognise when a mistake has been made and taking the appropriate action. Invariably, covering up errors only compounds the problem for the learner, quite apart from important questions relating to patient safety and being fair to peers and colleagues.

9. *Build in a system of recognising exceptional or even sound professionalism; this helps to ensure that a balance of positive and negative measures is there to support*

the development of professionalism among learners. Negative models can lead to negative attitudes and behaviours; it is all too easy to focus on problems without giving sufficient thought to the positive side of the equation, such as rewarding excellence in professionalism.

10. *Implement a system of formal sign-off on professionalism at the end of the education period. Ideally, both the learner and the institution should generate this together, reflecting the joint responsibility.* 'Being professional' means more than simply not getting into trouble. Giving recognition to students and trainees when they have met the agreed criteria for assessment in professionalism means that professionalism issues have higher visibility, and hence a higher profile in people's minds.

Case summaries

Case number	Student/trainee	Country	Description
1	Foundation doctor	UK	SE is found to be using drugs on the weekend, which affects her performance in the hospital, especially on Monday mornings (*see* p. 69).
2	Final-year medical student	UK	TW uses and sells nitrous oxide recreationally at a party; the media pick up the story and the student is dismissed from the school (*see* p. 72).
3	Foundation doctor	UK	RP goes through a bad period, during which time he receives a prison sentence for using cannabis; he 'settles down' and wants to be allowed to resume training (*see* p. 76).
4	Resident	US	RD begins to look unwell, and recent erratic performance is eventually linked to her husband's terminal illness; 'stress' leads her to write prescriptions for her own use (*see* p. 79).
5	Second-year medical student	US	DA is convicted of a serious drug crime; the school seeks to support a student in difficulties, but it is legally constrained and must deal with the lack of professionalism (*see* p. 82).
6	Junior resident	US	PW has repetitive absences from work; following interventions from the programme director, he successfully undergoes remediation (*see* p. 85).
7	Resident	US	KP is highly rated for her clinical performance but is repeatedly accused of unprofessional interactions, mostly by female colleagues (*see* p. 89).
8	Resident	US	JD abruptly decides to leave the programme for personal reasons that he is reluctant to disclose; he acts in breach of his contract, leaving co-residents to cover his clinical responsibilities (*see* p. 93).
9	Resident	US	SN has angry and emotional outbursts directed at nurses and medical students; when interviewed, he claims to be a whistle-blower (*see* p. 97).

Case number	Student/trainee	Country	Description
10	Junior resident	US	TI is a foreign-born trainee with significant research experience, but his training is marked by negative interactions with fellow trainees and poor performance on routine clinical tasks (*see* p. 101).
11	Junior resident	US	PM is accused of lying and other unprofessional behaviours; when challenged, she threatens to expose the programme director about a secret relationship with another resident (*see* p. 105).
12	Foundation doctor	UK	LT is a foreign-born trainee who covers up mistakes that he makes in the hospital; cultural attitudes seem to be behind the case, making it sensitive for the school to handle (*see* p. 109).
13	Final-year medical student	US	AY has an unexplained absence for an exam; he claims that his attention deficit hyperactivity disorder is a mitigating factor, but he failed to notify the school about this in advance (*see* p. 113).
14	Foundation doctor	UK	TP has negative interpersonal interactions due to autism; his clinical supervisor questions why he was allowed to graduate (*see* p. 116).
15	Third-year medical student	US	CA steals equipment from the hospital; he claims he needs it for his wife; eventually he has psychiatric assessment but he is never punished for the theft (*see* p. 120).
16	Medical student	NZ	JB is boastful about his sexual activities; lapses in professionalism occur, and it comes to light that he has relationship difficulties that could be linked to a mental health disorder (*see* p. 127).
17	Final-year medical student	AU	FH shows poor performance on a clinical exam; long-standing psychiatric problems are not being properly managed; the regulator is informed of breaches in professionalism, which spell an end to FH's career goals (*see* p. 130).
18	Medical student	NZ	MC becomes overly close to a patient, and she keeps important clinical information from the team; a mentor is appointed, at which point psychiatric issues begin to emerge (*see* p. 134).
19	Final-year medical student	AU	DZ fails an exam, which he claims is because of a previously undisclosed mental illness; he brings in a family lawyer to challenge what he claims is 'unfair discrimination' (*see* p. 136).
20	Medical student	NZ	MW assaults a female classmate; the following year he is caught falsifying work; after stern warnings about any repetition, he is eventually expelled, although the second incident is not related to the first (*see* p. 138).

Case number	Student/trainee	Country	Description
21	Final-year medical student	NZ	AB has frequent absences and episodes of dishonest behaviour; he is always charming and polite to staff, but he declines the offer of a mentor and has to repeat the year (*see* p. 141).
22	Second-year medical student	AU	SD is a poorly performing student, and while repeating a year in school, he continues to break rules, enlisting his uncle to sign off on clinical work; SD is not the only one being unprofessional (*see* p. 143).
23	Third-year medical student	AU	BJ is having a relationship with an administrative officer who works in the student assessments office; students become suspicious about alleged unfairness, and the situation becomes increasingly complex (*see* p. 146).
24	Medical student	NZ	JC has a medically unexplained illness that causes her to miss significant amounts of class time, including clinical requirements; patterns of frequent absence continue after graduation (*see* p. 149).
25	Third-year medical student	AU	TS is reported to the medical school by an affiliated hospital for a vague episode that occurred in the operating room; it appears that he may be being made a scapegoat for the behaviour of one of the senior surgeons (*see* p. 152).
26	First-year medical student	AU	YM refuses to have her required vaccinations because of family beliefs in homoeopathy; this prevents her progress into the clinical years, and she eventually decides to transfer to another school (*see* p. 156).
27	Medical student	NZ	AD is reported by a member of the public to be using marijuana and to own guns; issues arise about how the school should respond; he leaves the course, saying he no longer wants to pursue a career in medicine (*see* p. 159).
28	Medical student	AU	ME oversteps competency boundaries and gets involved with local politics during an elective rotation in a developing nation, claiming that one weekend 'he ran the hospital on his own' (*see* p. 162).
29	First-year medical student	AU	DP is older than his fellow classmates and takes on undue responsibility during a clinical elective in a developing nation; the school investigates his unprofessionalism, but some blame rests with the school (*see* p. 165).

Index

CPD with Radcliffe

You can now use a selection of our books to achieve CPD (Continuing Professional Development) points through directed reading.

We provide a free online form and downloadable certificate for your appraisal portfolio. Look for the CPD logo and register with us at: www.radcliffehealth.com/cpd

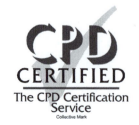

CPD CERTIFIED
The CPD Certification
Service
Collective Mark